Designing Your Perfect Dental Practice

Foundations of Clinical Success

Jay M. Hislop, D.D.S.

DESIGNING YOUR PERFECT DENTAL PRACTICE

Foundations of Clinical Success

Dental Communication Unlimited, P.O. Box 6405, Santa Maria, CA 93456
(805) 937-8711 • FAX (805) 937-3035 • E-Mail: sops@fix.net •
Website: http://www.sops.com

Portions of this book are available on computer disk, in either IBM/ compatible or Macintosh formats. Please contact DCU for details.

Other dental books available from DCU:

Standard Operating Procedures for All Dentists
Standard Marketing Procedures for All Dentists
Specialized Standard Operating Procedures for Pediatric Dentists
Specialized Standard Operating Procedures for Periodontists
Specialized Standard Operating Procedures for Endodontists
Specialized Standard Operating Procedures for Oral Surgeons
Specialized Standard Operating Procedures for Orthodontists
Risk Management for Dentists
Get Paid for Your Services: Simple, Sensible Payment Arrangements That Work!

ISBN 0-910167-55-9 (Cloth Bound)

Designing Your Perfect Dental Practice

Table of Contents

DESIGNING YOUR PERFECT DENTAL PRACTICE

Table of Contents: Standard Operating Procedures

All 26 SOPs listed above are available on computer disk for purchasers of Dr. Hislop's ***Designing Your Perfect Dental Practice***. Send $18 (tax and shipping included) to D.C.U. To help us send the appropriate disk, please indicate whether it will be used on an IBM/compatible or Macintosh computer. (See ordering instructions on the last page of this book—or call 800-563-1454.)

Jay M. Hislop, D.D.S.

Jay M. Hislop lives with his wife and two daughters in California, where he is the owner and consulting director of the Echelon Consulting Group, an innovative practice management consulting company. Dr. Hislop's company specializes in dental practice analysis, practice operations, strategic planning, time management, goal setting, and quality of life issues. He also has experience and expertise in the area of practice sales, mergers, group practice formation, and retirement transitions.

A 1978 graduate of the U.C.L.A. School of Dentistry, with General Practice Residency at Valley Medical Center of Fresno, he has been in public health practice as the founding Dental Director of the Battlefords Indian Health Centre in North Battleford, Saskatchewan, Canada. He has also been an owner and general dentist in solo and group practices in Stockton, California. In his practice, Jay focused primarily on full-mouth reconstruction, periodontal prosthetics, and esthetic dentistry.

Jay has been active in continuing education and has attended most of the prominent programs on clinical dentistry and practice management. After completing the entire course of studies at the L.D. Pankey Institute for Advanced Dental Education in Key Biscayne, Florida, he was invited to join the faculty, and later, the Board of Directors of the Institute. Jay currently teaches courses at the Pankey Institute, addressing the anterior and posterior considerations of the full-mouth reconstruction case.

Dr. Hislop lectures on the subjects of quality care of practice management and administration, business operations, advanced communications, dental reconstruction and rehabilitation, and periodontal prosthetics. He has written and lectured on the subjects of the threat of managed care to quality practice and the issues of practice management, domestically and internationally, since 1980. He is active in organized dentistry, serving on a number of committees and as a member of various Boards of Directors. Jay was the president of his component dental society in 1998.

His first book, ***Designing Your Perfect Dental Practice:*** *Foundations of Clinical Success*, is published by Dental Communication Unlimited.

Acknowledgments

I would like to thank all the great people who helped me put these thoughts on paper: the selfless and insightful people on the staff, faculty and board of The Pankey Institute for Advanced Dental Education who helped me understand the value we create for our patients, and gently guided me to crystallize my thinking and consciously apply philosophy to my life and practice; Marsha Freeman, who encouraged me to get started writing this book; my editor and publisher, Gordon Burgett, who with great ease and humor provided the knowledge and expertise for the logistics of this project, offered incredible insight into the inner workings of the writing process, and kept me moving through new and unknown territory; Dr. Gary Baughman and Dr. Lyndon Low, who painstakingly reviewed the chapter on orthodontic communications; Dr. Fred Bunch and Dr. Nick Veaco, who cut, cauterized, advanced and reassembled the surgical communications chapter; Dr. Randy Gordon, who practically rewrote the periodontal communications chapter; Dr. Irwin Becker, my long time friend, mentor and teacher, who provided much of the personal inspiration that led to this application of philosophy; Christian Sager, a fearless friend who has provided practical business guidance, no-nonsense planning, applied philosophy and future focus for me for many years; Dr. Richard Green, who challenged me to develop my understanding of human behavior with the same commitment that I made to technical training, and encouraged me to find ways to give back to the profession; pre-publication reviewers, including Dr. Tom Dawson, Dr. John Kois, Dr. Lucinda Lyon, and Dr. John Muller; my personal instructors and fellow faculty members at the Pankey Institute on whom I bounced these ideas before committing them to paper; the clients, friends and personal acquaintances who may find elements of their own story in my tale of the composite "Steve"; my friends who have been with me through the process to comment and offer encouragement; my wife, Gail, who never loses faith in me no matter what detour my life takes, or abyss I ask her to leap into with me, and my daughters Jenny and Kristen, who really are the best two kids ever, quite happy to accompany their dad into the “Fire Swamp" and other adventures of life, and who display maturity and grace beyond their years.

Cover design by Bruce-Paul Scott of Scott Graphic Design
(E-mail: bpscott@bpscottdesign.com)

Introduction

ACHIEVING YOUR DREAM

Do you remember the goals you had in dental school? Have you achieved the life you used to dream about? How many of us ever get there?

Tough questions, I know. But if you believe there is a better world in your imagination than the one in which you actually live, and you want to make it a reality, then this book is for you. It will give you some answers to those important questions about how to achieve your dreams in your practice and your life.

On a recent poll of dentists, over 50 percent said they would not select the profession of dentistry, should they have the opportunity to live their lives over again. Less than 30 percent said they were highly satisfied with their profession. Isn't this a sad commentary? Yes, but not the end of the story!

Most of the anxiety dentists feel has a familiar source—stress. Ask any dentist if he or she can name two things that will solve *most* of his or her problems, and nearly every one will have the same answer. "Help me find more patients and reduce my stress!" Or, "get rid of managed care and reduce my stress!" Or, "get this staff working *with me, not against me,* and reduce my stress!" "Lower my overhead and reduce my stress!" Stress is always the common denominator. Why should that be? We work in environments of our own creation; we provide helpful services to our fellow humankind, earn an enviable living, and enjoy enormous social and professional respect.

The answer is simple. 1) There is no longer the stable, predictable environment that once existed in our profession. 2) Dentists have lost control of their professional and practice lives. 3) Picture the typical dentist, trying to maintain a professional demeanor in the face of the pressures we all feel today!

Practice management is a chore; it seems to yield far too little return on investment in many dentists' minds. Practice overhead expenses are going crazy, rising at more than double the rate of inflation, and fees are under huge downward pressures from consumers and third parties. Patients are now "clients" at best, or "consumers" at worst, demanding accommodation of days and times. They're ferocious too, in their expectations of perfect results.

Of course there is OSHA, the CDC, your State Board, CE requirements, even Environmental Safety regulations, and soon waterline sterility and standards for sewage effluent coming from your office. Insurance companies are positioning themselves to be the primary care providers of all health care as soon as market forces allow. The result is either a severe erosion of the dentist's income or a changing pattern of practice to increase the number of days and hours worked just to keep up.

Loss of control causes the dentist to focus on the next problem, on the daily crisis, reacting to the situation and the environment until burnout occurs. Yet this elusive idea of a controlled professional life in dental practice remains alive in the minds of most dentists as a viable dream.

The dream can be attained! It's simple in concept and can be accomplished with sustained effort and commitment. Decide what you wish for yourself, your family, your staff and your patients. Then make it happen according to your own design. This book tells you how.

Let's begin by introducing you to a friend of mine…

Chapter 1

ONE DENTIST'S STORY

Dentists share a misconception. The misconception is that we somehow are gifted enough to create, manage and succeed at the very complicated and dynamic enterprise of dentistry without any training or expertise. Yet dentists come in all kinds of packages, and they bring their skills and weaknesses to the practice every day. Each dentist's practice is a reflection of that skill set he or she brings to work.

If the dentist is well organized, so will be the practice.

If the dentist is poorly organized, so will be the practice.

If the dentist has poor communication skills, the practice will not have a clear message that is conveyed to the public.

If the dentist is motivated solely by money, his or her staff will be greedy as well.

If the dentist is lazy and avoids unpleasant tasks, letting them build to crisis proportions, his or her staff will also procrastinate.

If the dentist is interested in the quality of care, the staff will be too.

If the dentist finds the *enterprise* of dentistry fascinating and challenging, and makes a study of small business management, the practice will be well managed.

I met Steve MacPearson, D.D.S., after he was in practice for nine years. Steve gets up each morning with high hopes for the day. After nine years in college and dental school, and another nine in practice, Steve feels like he should be in the peak years of his practice life. Yet at the end of each day he sits at his desk, defeated. He has a good practice, not what he would like it to be, but it has provided him with a living and many of the trappings of the successful health professional. He has not created a business. Nor has he created a professional life. He has created a personal job, and one that has begun to consume him.

"I went into dentistry because it offered me a chance to be my own boss and have a career in the sciences," Steve told me. "I was really a good student. I even thought about going into medicine for a while when I was in college. But I felt that the life of a physician was too demanding, and I really like to sail more than anything."

Steve was a high school record holder in four swimming events, was his high school valedictorian, and went to college on a swimming scholarship to one of the top universities in the country. While he was an undergraduate he took up sailing, joined the sailing club and became an exceptionally accomplished sailor.

"I really had very little time in college to plan my future," he said, gazing out the window to the bay over the stack of charts on his desk. "Yet I think this was a very good choice for me, knowing my aptitude for science and all. Do you realize how few jobs there were for science majors when I graduated in '83? Most of my friends and frat brothers went on to get a masters or something. Some of them are teaching; one is a college professor. A whole bunch of them are lawyers. The ones who were in the sciences and didn't pursue a professional career in medicine, dentistry, or teaching are not working in the sciences now. Some of my close friends wanted to work in an environmental science or resource job, or for Jacques Cousteau or someone like that. But there were more life sciences grads than dolphins left to study when I graduated. I only know of one who is actually working in the field. I think he's a forest manager.

"So when I went to see my advisor about careers, he suggested I consider dentistry. I had never even thought about dentistry before, other than being a dental patient as a kid. I had braces when I was a freshman in high school and hated every minute of it. I thought the girls wouldn't like a guy with braces, even though a lot of other kids had them. But I looked into it, even visited my family dentist when I was home on a break. Dr. Jennings was really enthusiastic about what he did. I was impressed with that, especially since he seemed to still really like what he was doing. He was even much older than my Dad, who was always complaining about his job. What I didn't realize was that old Doc Jennings was the last of an era. He worked virtually alone in a small office, probably with almost no overhead, and had earned and kept a small fortune many years before my visit with him.

"The next thing I knew, I was signing up for the DAT and applying to dental schools. Once I began that process, all my energy was focused on *getting in* to a good school. I never really questioned why, or if it was the correct choice after that."

I looked at Steve's diploma hanging over his desk. "You went to a great dental school," I said.

"Yes it is great, and I did very well there. I was in the top of my class, and actually enjoyed my dental studies. I think it prepared me very well for the clinical side of things. But it was very expensive, and I still am paying off some of my loans."

Steve was quiet for a moment.

"But you know, Jay, I'm really not very happy with the way things have turned out for me," he said, glancing my way. "I expected so much more. I don't know if I feel betrayed, but it seemed like this would be a lot more rewarding than it has turned out to be! Nobody in college—not my counselors or professors—had any idea about the profession they were steering me toward. Their knowledge was based mostly on their own personal experiences with their dentists. They really have no true knowledge of the profession and its challenges. It seems so trivial, but I guess I feel misled. Even the dental schools did nothing to help me understand what I was getting into."

He began to shuffle some of the mail on his desk. There was an enormous stack of journals and newsletters mixed with dozens of unopened envelopes. Even some patient charts were in the pile. The latest issue of *Dental Economics* was open to page 39.

You'll be hearing more about Steve as the book unfolds. Many dentists share similar difficulties putting it all together. The clinical side of things is often the easiest, because that is where our training is the most complete. The assumption among university professors and deans is that the quality of student who enters and completes dental school is a person who can "figure out" the rest of the problems and challenges of private practice. I have even heard the academic's excuse that dental students have no interest in learning practice management, so the deans and committees have not pushed it in the curriculum. Having been a dental student, I can attest to the fact that a great deal of the curriculum does not interest the students. But you sit there and learn it anyway. Nothing learned in dental school has as great an impact on a doctor's life, if he or she is in private practice, as the lessons learned from whatever resource about practice management.

Dentists are not clones of one another. There is no "typical" dentist, although we do share a lot in common. All happy dentists, however, are alike in several respects. They love their profession, and they have achieved economic success according to their own personal definition. Their lives are in balance. They are not consumed by their own practice. The practice is simply an important function in a balanced life, perhaps an element of great importance, but not the sole defining characteristic of the dentist's self image. Family, friends, spiritual life, recreation, intellectual pursuits, community activities, and much more are the elements and components of the lives of balanced dentists.

A prominent university dental school recently offered to its faculty the opportunity to enroll in graduate studies leading to an MBA, with instruction provided on site at the dental school. About 20 of the faculty enrolled. I wonder if this group includes any of the same faculty that have prevented a serious study of business management in the dental school. A dentist should not have to return for two years of graduate study and obtain an MBA in order to run a small business. Yet that may be the message in this faculty example. These "experts" in dental education themselves feel incapable of instructing the students in the business application of their clinical skills to make a profit, feed their families, send their kids to college and retire.

Dental practices are small businesses. The theories of small business management are very accessible, and dentists certainly have the aptitude and intellect to perform the duties of a small business owner/manager. That is not to say that small business is simple or effortless. Over 80 percent of all small business start-ups fail in five years. Dentists are far more successful at survival than that grim statistic. Yet dentists could be far more successful in the prosperity they derive from their efforts in small business if they would take it upon themselves to be as complete an expert about their *business enterprise* as they are about their *clinical profession.* This book is one component of a personal quest each dentist must begin in order to understand all the fundamental principles of the management of a private practice. It is not a comprehensive guide to practice management.

The following chapters will teach you the fundamentals of dental *enterprise* design. Steve will help illustrate the problems, and I'll help illuminate the solutions. It's up to you to implement the knowledge in your own life and dental practice.

Chapter 2

YOUR PREFERRED FUTURE IN DENTISTRY

"Actually, things seemed to be working better a few years ago," Steve said. "I had a practice that was about 30 percent larger than today with better organization. Now I'm having trouble making ends meet."

"What caused such a dramatic change?" I asked.

"I had a receptionist that was really incredible," he replied. "She did *everything*. There was nothing really for me to worry about. She kept the schedule busy, made the payment arrangements, sent the bills, collected the money, even hired my assistants—you name it she did it. Nina was the best receptionist I ever had."

"Why is she gone?"

"That was very hard for me to accept," Steve began. "Nina came on as a chairside assistant when I bought the practice. The previous receptionist, Eloise, had been with the former owner for many years and wanted to retire, but she was willing to stay on for about a year to help train her replacement. I knew nothing about all the management stuff. During that time Nina came on. She sort of did two jobs—front part time and back part time. Eloise complained that she was not learning 'the way we do things' but Nina felt the front desk was old fashioned. So I stayed out of it. When Eloise left early, I moved Nina full time to the front where she stayed for seven years."

"And she left two years ago?" I asked.

"Yes. That's when this place fell apart," he replied. "Looking back, it's pretty clear that she intended to leave for some time but didn't tell me. She started calling in sick by leaving a message with my answering service and we couldn't reach her by telephone. She did this several times over a few weeks. I think she was looking for another job. Then one day she left a message that she was quitting. Just like that. No notice or warning."

"I really had to scramble to fill in the gaps. I had to learn the computer system and all the little procedures that go on at the front. It was chaos for weeks. My other assistants were no use because they had only chairside training and no interest in taking 'Nina's' job."

"Do you know why she was unhappy?" I inquired.

"I got a hold of her later to find some addresses for insurance companies and to locate my bank statements. She said I didn't listen to her and didn't pay her enough for all the work she did here," he replied. "She wouldn't discuss it."

"So when did you get things straightened out?" I asked.

"Never!" he exclaimed. "We're still dealing with the aftermath of her exit. Both of the assistants she hired quit a few weeks after she did. It was almost as if they were mad at me for *her quitting*. My production fell and hasn't recovered. I've had problems hiring good staff. The whole practice just seems different."

"It's clear I was overly dependent upon her to run this place. But I never realized how good of a job Nina did because I didn't know *what she did*," he went on. "I haven't been able to find a person with her skills to take her place."

"How have you managed to get along?" I asked.

"Poorly," he replied. "I don't know if it will ever be the same. In a way, I'm hoping to just keep it small and see if I can make a profit so I don't ever have to suffer another decline like this one."

"Can you do anything to help me?" he asked. "Or is it too late?"

I had quite a bit of data on Steve's practice from a previous questionnaire so I was able to offer a partial answer: "It's not too late. But it will mean starting over again in a way. The practice has to be reinvented from the bottom up. It needs to have design and direction, a committed staff, an involved owner who participates, and much more..."

* * *

Steve's response to his situation is common. Many dentists try to *return to a former, usually smaller and more comfortable condition* when they find themselves in time of crisis. They do not have a clear mission, a philosophy of practice or a training manual to give to a new employee to get her up to speed fast. They want the practice to be "quit-proof" by having no person's absence cause so much turmoil. Unfortunately, this prevents the development of an organization that is equipped to handle change. Then when some other problem comes along, like a change in the insurance industry, the practice is unable to adapt.

Steve was managing a declining business. He had no hope for any meaningful growth and his profits were nearly non-existent. His wife was showing up at the office daily to get the day's receipts for a bank deposit. Nobody was tracking expenses. It was a busy practice ready to implode.

I had a lengthy discussion with Steve on the reasons he went into dentistry, his hopes and aspirations. We discussed his disappointments and perceived failures. Together we then sketched a mental picture of how Steve's "perfect practice" would look. For the first time in our short acquaintance I saw him really animated and enthusiastic. It is truly amazing what the imagination can do for a person's emotions.

I left Steve with some homework to do—the materials that appear in the next section.

Give it a try yourself. Even if your situation seems less grim than Steve's. The best situation can always be improved.

YOUR FUTURE OPTIONS IN DENTISTRY

Dentistry is a tough job. (As if you didn't know.) Dentists spend their days in awkward, uncomfortable positions, actually risking their own personal health, working in small, dark, steamy spaces on patients who are often ungrateful. To make matters worse, they provide a service most people claim they would avoid at all costs if possible. Not a very pretty picture is it?

Yet this profession literally attracts some of the best and brightest American college youth. They enter dental school with hopes and aspirations to achieve great things in a distinguished and respected profession. Each dental student has a unique story. Each one is fueled by various motivators from nobility to greed. Yet there are common themes that run through the student community and carry over to professional life.

Why did you choose this profession? Why are you a dentist? The fact is dentists do have much in common. Dentists share so many behavioral traits that during seminars it is easy to get groups of dental assistants and office staff people laughing by using humorous anecdotes about dentists. They always recognize their boss. Dental supply reps have their own hidden underground of unflattering humor and dark critical commentary about dentists. We are, for better or for worse, the product of our educational and professional training and experience.

If you are reasonably typical, you are in dentistry for many reasons common to us all. You had an aptitude for science and math. Your major in college was probably biology, other life sciences, chemistry, math or engineering. Less likely is a major in the liberal arts. You had a high GPA and scored high on the DAT. For many, that DAT score is the deciding element—evidence that their personal convergence of aptitude and interest is the dental profession. Many have had counseling in high school or college that led to a careful, rational decision to enter the dental profession. Others had a family member, personal dentist or friend who offered information, role modeling and encouragement to become a dentist.

Next, there was opportunity. The undergraduate position you attained allowed you the freedom to choose any number of professional or vocational directions. But dentistry is exclusive. Not everyone who has the desire gets to attend dental school. And you were one of the few who met all the criteria. So with aptitude and interest on your side, good grades and DAT scores and a reasonable desire, all that was left was the opportunity. Acceptance to a dental school, perhaps even the one of your choice, sealed your fate.

But what was really important was your desire. The motivation to spend yet another four years of your life to attain another degree was the real character trait that we all truly share. The desire was created by the very limited information about the profession that we have as a youth or a student in college. The profession is truly a calling. Each prospective dental student has an image of the life of a dentist in mind. The image has certain benefits and features. Freedom, financial prosperity, vocational independence, helping others, professional and community respect, working in applied science, providing a needed service, enthusiastic and helpful staffs, clean and efficient work environments, happy patients who love you, and various other factors attract and motivate the aspiring dentist. Seldom does the image include any elements or notions of striving, financial risk and responsibility, stress, work overload, and management or communication problems. Never does it include the kind of personal and professional malaise, apathy and burn-out we witness in nearly half of our colleagues who feel that they never quite get the job right.

Satisfaction in dentistry is not high. In most recent surveys of dentists, fewer than 50 percent would choose dentistry again. Mind you, this is very typical of surveys in all professions so part of these reflect the general malaise and dissatisfaction our society is experiencing as a whole. A recent survey of management workers in American corporations revealed only 35 percent felt secure in their jobs, and fewer than 50 percent would choose to work where they were presently working if they felt there was an option. This fact doesn't let us off the hook, however. We owe it to ourselves, and to our families, and to our patients to seek happiness in this profession.

So the important question you must first ask is: "How much do I want this life?" The fact that there is a significant percentage of dentists who *are* satisfied and feel *greatly rewarded* by their calling should bring hope to the entire profession. This book is for those who would like to achieve the level of satisfaction contained in their image of benefits and features that attracted them to the profession in the first place. Practical solutions are available. They can be incorporated into the routine of the dental practice in tangible ways that allow for the establishment and growth of a dynamic *and special* dental practice.

Is there a future in dentistry?

A few years ago, in the mid-1970s, Avrom King proposed a theory that dentistry would eventually stratify, and various tiers would emerge that would house distinctly different modes of dental practice. The various tiers would be primarily defined by two elements: 1) quality of care, and 2) the economic model under which the typical practice operates in each tier. The tiers are no longer theory. Dentistry has stratified. The tiers are not exactly as Dr. King envisioned them, so I have taken the liberty to define them as I see them...

The Pigeons

On the bottom tier are the capitation providers. I call these "Pigeons" because pigeons are kind of a land-based bottom feeder that only *looks* like a bird. Too short winged and pudgy to fly very well, they fly as little as possible. They prefer to walk along the ground, pecking at the sidewalk dust, knowing that by pecking enough of it some of it will be nourishing. They are dependent upon the urban environment for food and housing. Really just a feathered rat, they have no apparent useful purpose in the ecosystem, except opportunistic scavenging.

Like pigeons, capitation practices are really opportunistic scavengers. Really only giving the outward appearance of a dental practice, the pigeon practice is the home of the greediest of our profession. Economically they are based upon the premise that if they pick up enough contracts, some of them will be profitable. Since the capitation plans are typically underfunded, the doctors must "peck at" the patients. The unfortunate result of capitation contracts is that the doctors benefit from having as few of their contracted patients as possible seek or receive treatment. These practices are dependent upon urban environments to sustain a huge number of unsuspecting patients.

Don't underestimate the power of this trend. Capitation practices have the most aggressive marketing patterns, trying to achieve a visible place in the community. Unfortunately, employers have shown little concern about the *quality* of the benefit packages they offer employees. Employers are too often motivated only by costs. Capitation contracts offer the *promise* of a dental benefit for a *very cheap* price. This is understandably attractive to large urban employers, who may then offer the "benefit" to their employees. Quality is impossible for an employer to measure. And the designers of these capitation plans have done a clever end-run around the quality issue and turned it to their benefit. They include extensive "quality assurance" programs in their marketing proposals that appear to the lay person as a real assurance of practical quality. Price and quality in one package—how can you beat it? It is a temptation that many employers cannot resist.

Fortunately, capitation practices are somewhat self-limiting. The market has grown steadily to about 15 percent of the total pre-paid insurance market but has had problems making serious inroads outside of the major urban centers. It will probably peak with about 30 percent of the *total* dental marketplace and have the most major impact in the urban centers like Los Angeles. There other forms of practice will be increasingly difficult because of the price competition from well marketed *"Pigeon Practices."* Strategies to compete must begin to increase in sophistication, particularly in the areas of hospitality and marketing, in order to survive.

The Shorebirds

The next tier is a familiar practice type. This is the all-insurance retail practice. I call these "*Shorebirds*" because they are dependent upon one type of environment and one food source. They are seen in great abundance along the two coasts, but less in the interior. They are really very good fliers, but they are susceptible to environmental change, and this weakness can bring sudden death from relatively minor environmental changes. Some are quite small and agile, and others are large and ponderous.

The *"Shorebird Practice"* is totally insurance funded. It may be a combination of capitation, PPO, DMO and indemnity insurance in some ratio. The smaller, more agile practice will be largely indemnity funded and be represented by a killdeer or a willet. The larger, more ponderous will be largely capitation, represented by an albatross or pelican. They are in low to middle rent retail locations in strip centers and lower end shopping malls. This is probably the riskiest type of practice to have. It is not subject to much control by the owner. The practice will rise and fall on the tides of the insurance economy.

Having no effective internal controls, the owner of a *"Shorebird Practice"* is dependent upon the whims of the cumulative management decisions of various insurance company middle managers. It is impossible to effectively market, because your marketing target may or may not participate in one of your plans. It is unrewarding financially because you do not have any control over your fees. It is unrewarding professionally because the doctors don't have control over their patients' treatment plans. This is truly a doctor caught in an oil spill by drifting without a rudder through difficult economic times without a plan or a direction. The *"Shorebird Practice"* will be about 50 percent of the future dental practices, and represents about 20 percent of practices today. But each one is individually unstable and vulnerable.

This vulnerability is precisely what the insurance industry set out to create. It puts them in control of your practice. Look at how medicine is practiced today. It is a direct result of insurance industry profiteering at the expense of patient care. These practices are the ones most susceptible to buy-outs by dental management companies. The former owners will then become a sort of indentured servant of the corporation, unable to leave because of equity held as stock in a perilous corporation and unable to quit because of covenants not to compete.

The Songbirds

The third tier that has emerged is the mixed fee for service and insurance practice. This is like a songbird. Songbirds are small and very adaptable. Various species live from the tropics to the arctic circle. They are quite familiar and common. Songbirds are particularly accomplished in filling a narrowly defined niche. Each one has a unique set of habits and characteristics including feeding, nesting and migratory patterns. They are extremely adaptable.

This tier is the most common of all our tiers today—probably 50 to 70 percent or so of all dental practices. But this is a shrinking tier. Ultimately this tier will hold only 15 percent of all dental practices. The problem is not the quality of care or the adaptability of the dentists. There are two factors leading to the steady erosion of this practice form. The changing nature of the dental pre-paid insurance industry is driving more practices into the *"Shorebird"* tier; and the failure of dentists to learn the importance of communications in their management and marketing strategies is causing employers and patients to fail to see a difference in the type of care they receive. The successful *"Songbird"* of the future will have to have a practice that is primarily fee for service, with indemnity insurance as a limited part of the mix.

The Eagles

Eagles are self-defined and self-sufficient. Their stature and power is undisputed. Masters of flight, they soar above the reaches of most other species. Yet they are rare and tend to be limited in their range.

"Eagle Practices" have become the preferred practice for quality dentists in the last decade or so. It is the type of practice where the doctor can focus best upon quality patient care and can deliver the most relationship-based level of care. This is the practice most prospective dentists dream about when they form their image of practice. Yet few are able to achieve this level of professional expertise, clinical mastery, communications sophistication, management skill and entrepreneurial success. These are the true masters of dentistry. These are the doctors who are able to craft a balance in their lives that allow for excellence in dentistry, management expertise, personal and professional fulfillment and economic prosperity. Does this mean none of their patients have insurance? No it doesn't. But it does mean the office is managed to provide quality patient care based upon the relationship with the individual patient, without allowing the insurance to dictate treatment. If there are third-party funds available to assist the patient, so much the better. But that money relationship is between the patient and the payer, and the doctor and his staff are not in that loop. These doctors do everything that they can to see that the patients' insurance companies are given all the information they need to pay the maximum allowed. But treatment is not dictated by the insurance company.

"Eagle Practices" are not the exclusive subject of this book. Certainly *"Songbirds"* can exercise considerable self-determination as well. The point is: Have you chosen? Or are you in your tier by happenstance?

You must decide!

Yes, each of us must decide. Each dentist must think about his or her career in dentistry like we've never thought before. If not, the entropy of the insurance industry will pull you to the lowest tier and your satisfaction with your profession and your life will be dismal. It is necessary to be aware and understand these trends in order to position yourself in the tier of your choice. Yes, *it is a matter of choice!* You always have the right to choose. The question is only whether you are willing to step up and pay the price to change from discontent to professional self-determination and satisfaction.

Dentistry has always offered the hope and possibility of personal financial prosperity. This is probably not the best motivation for entering the profession, but is certainly a factor in most prospective dentists' decisions, and a present goal for most practitioners. Casting one's fate to the whims of a fickle insurance economy cannot possibly yield professional fulfillment. When faced with forces too big to overcome and change, the answer is not necessarily to simply forfeit your self-determination and to acquiesce. Another choice is to find another direction, a new way to approach the problem.

Prosperity and professional satisfaction are not accidents. It is the result of careful and honest evaluation of your present situation and a vision of your preferred future. The emotional stress we all feel when those two things don't match can provide the motivation to make the changes from our current world to the preferred world of our vision.

Planning your preferred future

Successful careers are not the result of random events. We all know of practices that somehow rise above the level of others in the same community. There is more energy, more enthusiasm, more visible appearances and expressions of satisfaction in the practice. These practices are usually well respected in the community, and the patients receive a high quality level of care. The doctors who own these practices are comfortable with their lives and satisfied in their profession. How did they do it?

Satisfying practices are the result of careful design and planning. Planning is the one activity that can create growth in a direct and linear way, in the proper direction to fulfill one's goals. Simply setting a goal is not enough. Planning begins the process of creating change that yields the exact results to fulfill the vision originally created in the mind of the doctor.

In *Control Theory* by William Glasser, the process is referred to as "gap analysis." In this theory of planning for meaningful change, the planner draws three columns on paper. In the left column, write down all the attributes, features, and benefits of the quality world that you would like to achieve. In the right column, write down a corresponding description of the perceived world in which you find yourself today. The middle column is "the gap." It describes the behaviors that are yielding your current results. Use the gap to describe: 1) "What I do." 2) "What I think." 3) "What I feel," and 4) "What I experience physiologically."

When one has expectations that are not being met, the result is emotional and physiological discomfort. The way to move from emotional and physiological discomfort to emotional and physiological satisfaction and well-being is to complete the Gap Analysis. At that point, answer the following questions:

1. What is it precisely that I want? (The quality world of *Control Theory.)*
2. What am I currently doing to get what I want?
3. How is what I am doing working? (Or not working?)
4. What else can I do to get what I want?
5. *What will I do?*

Then begin to form the elements of a plan. A plan must have a clear and definable outcome, measurable in terms that are defined by the desired outcomes. To provide the bearings and direction for individual accomplishment, a plan must have these elements:

1. It must fulfill a defined need.
2. It must be simple and specific.
3. It must be attainable, realistic.
4. It must be clear, well defined and measurable.
5. It must be immediate, able to be implemented today.
6. It must be repetitive.
7. It must be contingent only upon individual behavior.

A plan must not assume that elements outside of your direct control will respond in specified ways in order to achieve your desired result. You cannot depend that others will respond in predictable ways according to your plan.

So what's next? Now that you have some idea of the forces at work in dentistry, and the need to have a clear plan, you can begin to design your own future. Let's take a look at the process in detail in the next chapter.

Chapter 3

DESIGNING YOUR FUTURE: "VISIONEERING" YOUR DENTAL PRACTICE

Steve and his wife, Eileen, were both from the San Francisco Bay area and went to a major university there, where they met. Their relationship became serious during Steve's senior year, and they married during his second year of dental school after Eileen graduated from the university. Eileen worked while Steve attended school, but they survived mainly on student loans. Even with his big student debt, Steve was able to arrange financing to buy a small practice in the expensive hill area near his home. When Eileen became pregnant, the couple decided to buy a house. Again they were able to find a mortgage lender. By then Steve's practice had grown significantly, and his income looked promising, though his debt was enormous and growing with the new mortgage.

Steve and Eileen quickly moved up through three different homes during the first nine years of his practice, two of them new ones in new developments. Each home represented a step up for Steve and his growing family. After their fourth child, they decided there would be no more babies. When I met Steve, Eileen was a full-time Mom; she had plenty to do with children ranging in age from one to seven.

Steve's work day is fairly typical of most dentists. As he heads out the door for his morning jog, he passes a few neighbors getting ready to face their day. Steve has maintained a very visible life in his city, attending most important community functions. He's a member of the Rotary Club—he's a past president and tries to present an appearance of success. As he jogs along, he thinks about his community contacts, realizing they have been responsible for most of his practice growth, and he ponders how much effort he has made to carefully maintain his professional image. As Steve runs past the houses on his suburban street, he sees others leaving for work.

"There goes Marty," he thinks to himself, "Poor sap *really* hates his job." Marty works as a personnel director in a major bank and has had to layoff more people than he has ever hired since the era of corporate mergers and downsizing began. Dealing with the effects of literally thousands of angry and hostile employees has really taken its toll. Steve thinks about the three times he has had to fire employees and shudders.

"I guess what I do is not so bad; I can't imagine having that many people hate me," he ponders. Steve recalls a shooting that occurred in the local branch of Marty's bank, and the weeks of turmoil in Marty's family that followed as Marty tried to deal with the aftermath among the employees.

"At least I'll never face that kind of crisis," he thinks.

Steve's house is a large two-story faux Tudor mansion overlooking a ravine well above the bay. He can see just a slice of the bay, shining in the distance from the corner window of his bedroom. It was the best view he and Eileen could afford, in what they hope is the last house they'll ever have to buy. Most of his neighbors are professional people or management-level employees of major corporations. It is a very affluent neighborhood.

"It was a big step to buy this house, but Eileen and I decided it was now or never, so we bit the bullet," he once told me. "It's been a struggle every month since then. Sometimes Eileen comes to the office to get the deposit so we can make our mortgage payment on time. But we've never been late, and things always work out so I don't worry about it, much."

As Steve rounded the curve of the hill he waved to Roger, who was waiting for him at the top of the curve.

"Hi Rog, how's it going," Steve greeted his running mate.

"Great, you?" Roger replied.

The pair run a daily 5.5-mile loop into the hills above their subdivision, meeting each day at the same place. Roger is the Dean of Graduate Studies at Steve's alma mater and is almost 15 years older than Steve. He is in much better shape than Steve, and they look nearly the same age. They met while jogging in the neighborhood two years ago and have been running partners ever since.

"Roger, how do you do it?" Steve puffed as they ran up the steepest grade in the loop. "You're already old and gray," Steve joked, "yet you kick my butt every day on this hill."

"Clean living, I guess," Roger joked back. "Actually, I was really overweight when I was your age. I think its a function of the stage of life I was in then—too much to do and not enough time. I decided when I made tenure to get back in shape, and it stuck. I guess dentists don't get tenure though, huh?"

Steve pondered this for a minute. "No, we just get rich," he lied.

"Yeah, I know," said Roger, "I saw Eileen's new Lexus in the driveway."

"Hey, that's *my* Lexus!" Steve protested, "Eileen drives the Caravan."

"Yeah, sure," Roger jabbed.

The pair ran in silence for a while.

"Roger, honestly, how do you stay in shape. I run with you every day. Obviously I eat a ton, and I know I should lay off the junk food, but *you* are *fit*!"

"Well, Steve, this is only my wake-up call. I have the university athletic facilities at my disposal, so I usually put in another hour at lunch, or right after work—swimming or playing basketball with some faculty guys," Roger replied.

"You sandbagger!" Steve protested. "I should have known you were working out on the side!"

"You're not in such bad shape, for a fat guy," Roger smiled, hoping Steve would take it as a joke.

Steve shot a glance at Roger, and realizing the joking banter said, "Yeah, I'm not so bad, compared to a lot of my friends. But I've been a lot better. You should have seen me in college."

"I did, you being a swimming star and all. You just didn't know *me* then. Probably a good thing. I was a mean professor," Roger replied.

"Yep, Olympic dreams and Pac 10 ability," Steve quipped.

* * *

Steve thought for a moment. Then he said, "One thing for sure, I'd be in better shape."

"I would also like to be out of debt, and not have the stress on my family finances that I feel now. I'd like my work days to be smooth and more predictable. And I'd like a committed staff who care more about the practice and the patients than about their petty grievances."

"You mean care about the practice like you do?" I asked.

"Yes, and are willing to go the little extra step that it takes to really make things happen for people," he replied. "I'd really like to able to provide the kind of top level care that I think successful practices are going to have to provide to keep from getting taken over by managed care," he added. "I don't know how to do it, but I think only a few practices are going to be private, fee-for-service based in just a few more years."

"I really want to feel good about the care we are providing our patients, and maybe even feel that they appreciate what we do for them. I know I need to bring some of my clinical skills up to date, but that is a fun and rewarding challenge. What I don't know how to do is to get the practice *ready* for whatever it is we're facing. It is really hard to battle with things you don't fully understand. It all seems so much out of control."

"What about your family life?" I asked.

"Most of the problems Eileen and I have are financial. And time," he added. "I wish I had more time to spend with the kids. My oldest is starting to play baseball and soccer, and I haven't been able to be as involved as I would like to be. Plus we're always short of cash for our lifestyle, and we use credit cards a lot. We haven't begun yet to save for retirement, or college for that matter, and I really don't know where *that* money is coming from!"

"How about your recreation?" I asked.

"Well, I said I'd like to be a lot more fit. I run with this guy in the neighborhood who is a lot older than I am, and he's really in much better shape. I'd like to be like Roger when I'm his age, but at the rate I'm going I'll never get there," he replied. "I would like more time to sail, and to teach my kids how to sail. We don't do enough together as a family. There really isn't enough time, and the weeks go by so fast, it's hard to focus on some of this stuff."

"And your spiritual life?" I asked.

"We don't go to church very often anymore, though both Eileen and I were raised in the same faith and went to parochial schools. Our parents did a much better job with us than we're doing teaching our kids. It's all so much more complicated now than it was when we were kids," he lamented. "I just wish life were simpler."

"How do you feel about all of this?" I asked, knowing the answer I was about to hear, having heard it hundreds of times before.

"I *hate* it!" Steve thundered. "I feel frustrated, even *angry* that I can't have the things I'd like to have and live the life I think I deserve. I know it sounds selfish, but it isn't just about me, it's about my family, my patients, the *whole thing*. There is so little time for what's important to me! My practice consumes almost all of my emotional energy just dealing with the problems and all. I have very little left for everything else! Sometimes I feel like my life is like a heart in *ventricular fibrillation,* lots of pumping but no blood flowing anywhere."

"Nice analogy," I said. "Can I use that in my lectures?"

Steve smiled, "I guess I'm overstating the problem a bit, but I really am frustrated!"

*　　　　*　　　　*

Many dentists complain about a loss of control over their lives and practices. The forces of change that we just described along with the dentist's own lack of "visioneering" create practices and lives that are adrift, rudderless in the sea of change. Yet, most of us just want to "get to work." Seldom do we want to take the time to sit down and do the really hard stuff—planning. And the results are predictable.

We end up someplace we didn't intend to be. It is this very *intention itself* which we lack, not the ability to go where we want to go in our professional lives.

This chapter will give you the tools to simply and effectively create your personal vision for your practice and professional life. By the way, the same processes can be used to join with your family in a plan to create a vision you can share for your personal and family futures.

Creating a vision for your practice is much the same process as an architect would use to create a vision of a building. Though a building seems more tangible, sitting solidly anchored to the earth, it is really no more or less tangible than a dental practice. Think about it. The practice has a certain space it occupies, certain types of activities go on there, and certain people interact in various ways. It can be a wonderful place filled with service and success, or it can be a stressful place filled with confusion and disappointment. The choice is yours. You simply need to take the first few steps to *design* it.

Step 1—It is your world. Just imagine that.

The first step is often the hardest. But remember the old cliché: "Well begun is half done." Sit down in a comfortable place with a pencil and a big pad of paper. Visioneering requires a little of your time and all of your imagination, so try to have some time with no distractions. Go to your mountain retreat or to the coast if necessary, but don't postpone this beyond the next available weekend! Do it *now*! Once you set this book aside and say "Good ideas, I'll get to those sometime soon"—you're doomed to continuing your present uncharted path indefinitely.

"Personal," "Preferred" and "Chosen"; write those words down at the top of the page. This is the definition of a "visioneered" practice and life.

Now, imagine your perfect world. Think big. Don't limit yourself by the constraints you are experiencing in your present circumstances. Circumstances can be overcome in time. Designing a chosen life is only the first step, so don't get hung up with issues of possibility or impossibility. Time will take care of those kinds of issues. But do be realistic. If you want "money for nothing," then you will need to write a plan for financial independence, including a timetable. Your task at hand is to design your personal, preferred and chosen future.

Step 2—Elements of Your Chosen World

The purpose of this exercise is to create a set of elements that can be used to crystallize your thinking about your preferred future.

Here the sky is the limit. But to contain and direct your thoughts, think of your life as having four interrelated components that you must try to juggle and balance. L.D. Pankey described these areas like the points on a compass he called the "Cross of Life." This is an excellent way to organize your thoughts. The four areas are work, play, love, and worship. More information and detail about Pankey's philosophy of dental practice can be found in *A Philosophy of Dental Practice,* by L. D. Pankey and W. J. Davis. For our purposes of visioneering, let's take a look at each of the areas in turn:

A. **Work:** Your financial health begins with work and its rewards. Your vision of your dental practice must include a working plan to achieve your professional and financial goals.

There are many elements of your practice to consider as you design your future. To begin, you need only describe the basic elements of how your work life balances with the other three elements. Answer the following questions:

- How many days a week will you practice?
- Will you have a large or a small staff. How do you define this?
- How many patients are you comfortable seeing each day?
- What types of procedures do you really like doing?
- What types of procedures do you dislike enough that you would mostly refer if you had the choice?
- What are your major strengths and interests?
- Which of these would you like to develop and enhance?
- Describe the "feel" of your quality office setting.

How much income do you desire? (Net, take home salary and profit.)

How hard are you willing to work for it? (These two areas are very closely related. Don't make the mistake of visioneering unlimited income with little or no work and no time to make it happen.)

B. Love: Your family life, your social life and friendships

Much of this discussion is centered on the personal rewards of family and friendships. To help in crystallizing how this fits into a scheme of dental practice, work through the following questions and thoughts:

1. Are you married or do you intend to marry?

What are your criteria for a great relationship with your spouse? Here are some ideas to focus your thinking:

- My spouse runs the home, I bring home the bucks.
- My spouse must be the anchor that holds the family together, so I can focus on work.
- My spouse is a working partner in my business.
- My spouse supports my vocational activities emotionally by understanding my need to communicate my difficulties at work.
- My relationship is a partnership; it involves some interaction of both of our work lives.
- Work and family are to be kept separate.

Write a statement to describe your ideal marriage or relationship. Share this process with your spouse.

2. How do you see your role as a parent?

- No children ever!
- Somewhat active, but no primary parenting responsibilities.
- Very active, sharing and dividing parenting tasks equally with my spouse.
- My primary role in life. My practice must take a second place to my primary parenting role.
- I have no time for practicing dentistry

Write a statement describing your preferred role as a parent.

3. How do you view your friendships and community activities?

- My friends provide an interesting way to spend some of my free time.
- Friendships are very important.
- My friends sustain me, support me.
- I live for my friends.
- I balance my friendships and social activities well with my other life areas.

Write a brief statement about your preferred role in your community.

4. How do you see your role with your staff?

- As a commander, they will do what I say.
- As a leader.
- As a friend.
- As a lifelong companion in practice.

Write a statement to describe the preferred level of leadership and personal relationships you desire with your staff.

C. Play: Your recreation and avocations

The purpose of this section is to illuminate the importance of the role of recreation in your life. Many people live for something other than dentistry such as taking their family skiing or sailing, writing, painting. Whatever it may be, if that is true for you, be honest.

Remember, recreation is not simply time off to play. It should be a time of physical and mental renewal, allowing for continuous effectiveness and improvement in the other three areas of your life. Its importance must not be underestimated as you begin your preferred future.

- My favorite forms of recreation are:
- When I participate in _________, I feel:
    - ◊ Renewed and refreshed
    - ◊ Tired but invigorated
    - ◊ Tired and lethargic
    - ◊ Tired and frustrated
    - ◊ Frustrated and angry
    - ◊ Angry, injured, with expensive equipment wrapped around tree trunks
- I need to have more/less physical exercise
- I am/am not very healthy, fit, and not overweight
- I need more/less intellectual stimulation
- I need more/less time to play with my family
- I need more/less time to play with my friends
- I need more/less time alone

Write a paragraph about how you have experienced your recreation and avocation life in the past several years.

Write a statement that defines your recreation and avocation in your preferred world.

List your chosen avocation and recreation pursuits.

D. Worship: Your spiritual world

Here, a book about dental practice begins to tread on some risky territory. Obviously, volumes have been written since the dawn of man about this subject, and no claim will be made here of any answers. However, it is an element of your life that deserves enormous attention and reflection. Here are some thoughts to assist your visioneering:

- How do you worship?
- Is worship a part of your life?
- Do you take time each day to appreciate life?
- Do you pray or meditate?
- Are you at peace with the world around you and in your relationships with others?
- Are you making a contribution to humankind, and doing your part to make a more perfect world?
- Is your spiritual life assisting or interfering with the prosperity of your practice?
- Do you impose your religious beliefs upon others? Your patients?

If you can, write a statement of your personal religious philosophy.

Write a statement that describes the role of spiritual life in your preferred world.

Step 3—Your Personal Mission Statement

Now you have all the tools you need to write a personal mission statement. I know you've been through this before!

But now you have the tools to create a mission statement that actually serves you by providing the first brick in the foundation of your preferred future! Besides, it is really easy. So again, don't hesitate, just get on with it!

A. Begin with summaries of the four interrelated elements:

1. Summarize your thoughts on your work.
   - Write a brief statement of philosophy of why you are a dentist.
   - Write a brief statement of how your profession fits into the larger scheme of your life.
2. Summarize your thoughts on your roles in your family and friendships.
   - Write a brief statement about your attitudes and experiences of your best and most preferred relationships.
   - Think about how you would like to create this world.
3. Summarize your thoughts on recreation and avocations.
   - Write a brief statement of philosophy for this area.
4. Summarize your thoughts on worship.
   - Write a brief statement of philosophy here as well.

Here is an *example* of how this summary might look. Be careful not to simply use this one, since it is fictitious and a composite of many people. Yours will only work if you create it yourself.

1. I need to make a contribution to humankind. My work life must be rewarding both financially and emotionally. My most important goal in life is to be financially independent by age 65, so I will never burden my family. My workplace must be calm and not a source of stress.

2. My family is the most important part of my life. Yet I know our family would shatter if we didn't have economic security, so those elements must be balanced. I want to be a great father/mother for my kids and be very active in their lives. I am a faithful spouse and it is important for me to maintain this relationship forever. My friendships are important to me, but not as much as my family or my work. I see myself as a great friend to a few select people.

3. I once lived to ski (sail, fish, bicycle, knit, cook, read...). But now I see this must not be my defining principle. It was appropriate in my 20s, but now my life has taken other directions that are of my own design. These are yielding greater rewards. Therefore, recreational pursuits can no longer predominate in my life, and my recreational life needs to provide me the following:

    - A high level of fitness
    - Relaxation

- Fun
- Time with my family and friends
- Mental renewal
- Intellectual stimulation outside of dentistry

4. My spiritual life is the source of my strength and wisdom. It has been subjected to considerable neglect in recent years. In order to achieve my preferred future, my spiritual life needs some immediate attention.

    - I need to attend to my spiritual needs on a regular basis
    - I will take time each day to celebrate life
    - My attitude will be predominately positive
    - I believe I am a spiritual being having a life experience
    - I can contribute to the world just by being alive

B. Now write a Personal Mission Statement in a way that resonates for you. It may be a single sentence, a paragraph or two or even a poem.

Examples:

I believe I am here to:
Be a loving husband and father
Be the best dentist I can be
Enjoy my life
Worship God

My mission in life is to be creative. I have much to contribute to the world, and I feel that my purpose on earth is to find ways to contribute.

My mission is:
To foster understanding and promote good works
To give freely of myself and all I discover
To live in joy and harmony with the environment
To experience the miracle of the world

I am here to be the best dentist, father and friend I can be.

My purpose in life is to provide for my family. I am the one responsible for our economic well-being, the foundation of our existence. I will be diligent in my professional efforts in order to provide a comfortable and happy life for my family.

My purpose in life is to be humble and thank God for all existence. I want to do good works on the earth and to prove myself worthy of His blessings.

From Mahatma Ghandi:
Let the first act of every morning be to make the following resolve for the day:
I shall not fear anyone on earth.
I shall fear only God.
I shall not bear ill toward anyone.
I shall not submit to injustice from anyone.
I shall conquer untruth by truth.
And in resisting untruth, I shall put up with all suffering.

From Alfred Lord Tennyson:
To strive, to seek, to find, and not to yield

From William James:
To improve the golden moment of opportunity, and catch the good that is within my reach.

From *Ecclesiastes* 9:10
Whatsoever thy hand findeth to do, do it with thy might.

Now check back through your notes to be sure your personal mission statement mirrors to you the *essence* of your purpose in life. It need not restate every element; it must merely be able to *contain* them. If your mission statement contains the essence of your reflections in each of the four areas above, then move on. If not, try restating it another way until you are comfortable that it defines your essential purpose.

Step 4—Your Preferred World of Work

Now that you have a better view of the "big picture" of your life, we will revisit your dental practice. Your goal here is to articulate your quality world a bit more clearly.

1. How do you want to define your practice? Here are some examples:

    - Fee-for-service
    - Family practice
    - Cosmetic practice
    - Restorative or reconstructive practice
    - Relationship based practice

- Specialty practice
- Welfare
- Clinic
- Group
- Solo
- Exclusive

2. What do you want most from your practice?
3. What are your personal strengths?
4. What are your favorite tasks?
5. Your least favorite tasks?
6. Design your ideal day:
    - Beginning time
    - Number of patients
    - New patient exams
    - Consultations
    - Recalls and hygiene check-ups
    - Staff interactions
    - Telephone calls
    - Charting time
    - Production
    - Collections
    - Stress level
7. What do you want patients to say about you and your office?
8. What do you want your referring doctors to say?

Write a statement that clearly describes the features of your ideal dental practice. Include as much detail as possible about the pace, the type of dentistry, the stress level, the enjoyment, and the satisfaction you experience in this ideal practice. Think about characteristics of the staff you would choose to work with and the patients you would choose to serve.

Step 5—Your Professional Mission Statement

Now that you have a personal mission statement that is clear and true to you, it is a simpler task to write a *Professional Mission Statement.* This is also a personal document and will become one of the tools used later with your staff to produce a *Practice Mission Statement.* I know it may seem a bit much, but the lack of this foundation is the common denominator among nearly all the disappointed dentists of the world.

Your *Professional Mission Statement* is a simple statement that describes why *you* are in this profession. You may have chosen dentistry for entirely selfish reasons, and that is OK. Or you may be in it for entirely noble reasons. Whatever *your* reasons, they need to be crystal clear to you before you can move on.

The important questions to ask to prepare this statement are:

1. What do I want most from dentistry?

2. My favorite aspects of dentistry are:

3. I want my patients to remember me by:

4. If I could live my life over I would choose:

5. In five years I would like my practice to be:

6. In ten years I would like to be:

7. After all is said and done I am a dentist because:

Now, write a *Professional Mission Statement* that summarizes your findings above.

Examples:

I am a dentist because it is an easy way to make a lot of money.

My purpose as a dentist is to preserve the health of my patients.

My purpose is the pursuit of excellence in my dental practice; to provide to the best of my ability and talent dental services that create and restore function, comfort, esthetics and a sense of physical well-being for my patients.

From Dr. L.D. Pankey:

I made a commitment to myself. I would never take out another tooth as long as I lived...I did not know how I was going to do it, but I had decided to dedicate my life to saving people's teeth.

From Dr. H. Loren Miller:

If the central theme of the philosophy were to be addressed in a few words, it would be about a balanced life, a pursuit of excellence in all facets of the balance.

Step 6—Writing Your Practice Mission Statement

Writing the *Practice Mission Statement* is an exercise that must be completed with the participation of your staff. This is not a rehash of your Personal or Professional Mission Statements. It is a document that is the foundation for the structure, procedures, teamwork and communications that define the reality of your practice.

Ideally, each member of the staff should have a personal mission statement and professional mission statement of his or her own. This is difficult to achieve in many offices, and is not a requirement for success. But if you want to soar to the top of your profession and truly be an "eagle," give it a try. Give a copy of this chapter to each staff member before your practice mission workshop, and see if some of them are receptive to the idea of a personal mission and professional mission. They might surprise you. It will certainly give you an indication of who the really dedicated players are on your team. The author began this process many years ago, and numerous staff members over the years have expressed appreciation for being given a technique that helped them in their own lives and relationships. It has been very gratifying.

The practice mission is then written as a group exercise in usually two meetings. Prior to the first meeting, have the staff complete their own personal and professional mission statement, as well as the Mission Statement Questionnaire.

First workshop: Have each team member bring the completed questionnaire to the workshop. It may be wise to consider hiring a facilitator to assist with the process of mission writing. (Resources are available from various Certified SOP Consultants and can be reached by first contacting either the author at 1-800-799-5049 or D.C.U. at 1-800-563-1454.)

A. Write down on a flip chart key words and phrases each team member shares from his or her own questionnaire.
B. Try to have contributions from each team member.
C. Keep an open, non-judgmental atmosphere.
D. As a group, decide and agree upon a mission statement and a list of objectives.
E. If your team is very large, divide into two or three smaller groups to each come up with a mission, then come together and have a member of each group present a concept for final collaboration.

Second workshop: After the first workshop, have an assigned scribe bring the collaboration to a draft of the written document. Print copies and distribute them among the staff to read and ponder for a week or so. Then come back together for a second, usually much shorter session.

A. Invite comments about the mission statement.
B. Facilitate and collaborate changes or modifications that clarify, simplify or illuminate the draft.
C. Agree on a final form.
D. Celebrate the formulation of your mission.

After the workshop, print the final mission statement and distribute among the staff. It is also a good idea to have a larger version laser printed to post where the staff can see it daily.

Step 7— Updating the Mission Statement

The Practice Mission Statement is a collaborative creation of your entire staff. Of course, the staff changes with time as employees come and go. So periodically it is necessary to update the mission. Here's how to do it simply and easily:

A. Distribute the Mission Statement Questionnaire
B. Add the following supplemental questions:

1. What changes (if any) would you like to see to our Practice Mission Statement to have it relate more thoroughly to our current staff?
2. What should our objectives be for the coming year?

C. Hold a workshop to discuss, collaborate and *update* the Practice Mission Statement. This can be accomplished in one session. Do this annually even if you have experienced no staff changes.
D. Celebrate the ongoing accomplishment of your mission.

CONGRATULATIONS!

You have just completed the first and most difficult step in creating the practice of your dreams. You have created a *vision* of that practice and distilled it down to a succinct mission statement. This is the foundation for everything that follows.

In the next chapter, you will learn how to effectively and efficiently communicate your practice philosophy to your staff, your patients and your referral network.

MISSION STATEMENT QUESTIONNAIRE

[msquest.3]

1. What three things do I want most from our practice?

2. What are the major strengths of our practice?

3. Why do patients come to us?

4. Why do patients leave?

5. If I could change one thing about our practice it would be…

6. The favorite part of my daily routine is…

7. The least favorite part of my daily routine is…

Mission Statement Questionnaire/ 2

8. My ideal day...

	... would look like this:	... currently looks like this:
Total # of patients		
# of new patients		
# of recall patients		
Production ($)		
Collections (%)		
Start day (time)		
End day (time)		
Stress level		

9. I want our patients to say this about our practice...

10. I want our referring doctors to say this...

11. Words and phrases that best describe what I'd like our office to be like for each other and for our patients...

12. After all is said and done, I am in the dental profession because...

13. A mission statement I could be proud of and enthusiastically work each day to meet is...

Mission Statement Questionnaire/ 3

14. Objectives for our office:

    a. Patient service ________________________________
    b. Team work ____________________________________
    c. Financial ______________________________________
    d. Equipment _____________________________________
    e. Continuing education ___________________________
    f. Practice growth ________________________________
    g. Expansion _____________________________________
    h. Other ____

Supplemental Questions for Update Workshops:

15. What changes (if any) would you like to see to our Practice Mission Statement to have it relate more thoroughly to our current staff.

16. What should our objectives be for the coming year?

From *Standard Operating Procedures for All Dentists* by Marsha Freeman.

PERSONAL MISSION WORKSHEET

[permissn.3]

Desired Outcome: To complete a written personal mission statement that is the essence of your purpose in life and will provide the philosophical foundation for all areas of your life.

Measurement: A written document exists that you can update as necessary.

Steps:

1. Begin by imagining your perfect world. Make a list of key words and phrases that describe that world.

2. Record the elements of your "chosen" world in four interrelated but discreet areas:

   A. Work:

Write a description of your practice configuration using ideas from the text.

Include income desires.

Include work days and times.

   B. Love:

Write a statement to describe your ideal relationship. Share process with spouse or significant other.

Write a statement describing your preferred role as a parent.

Personal Mission Worksheet / 2

Write a statement to describe your desired role in community life.

Write a statement to describe your ideal friendship relationships.

C. Play:

Write a paragraph about how you have experienced your recreation and avocation life in the past several years.

Define recreation and avocation in your preferred world.

Now list your chosen avocation and recreation pursuits.

D. Worship:

Write a statement of your personal religious philosophy.

Write a statement that defines the role of your spiritual life in your preferred world.

3. Write the mission statement

A. Write four summary statements that are the essence of your preferred world of:

Work.

Personal Mission Worksheet / 3

Love.

Play.

Worship.

B. Write your <u>*Personal Mission Statement*</u> using as much space as needed.

PROFESSIONAL MISSION WORKSHEET

[profmiss.3]

Desired Outcome: To have a written professional mission that is the personal foundation for a dentist or dental staff member. It is the essence of why you are in the dental profession.

Measurement: A written document has been prepared by the individual doctor or team member.

Steps:

1. Think about a perfect or ideal day at work. Write down as many key words and phrases to describe that day. Use the text for ideas.

What do you want most from your profession?

What are your personal strengths, and how can these fit with your ideal practice?

What are your favorite tasks?

Your least favorite?

2. Design your ideal day:

Start time	________
Number of patients	________
New patient exams	________
Consultations	________
Recalls/Hygiene checks	________
Staff interactions	________

Professional Mission Worksheet / 2

Telephone calls	____________
Charting time	____________
Production	____________
Collections	____________
Stress level	____________

3. I want my patients to remember me by:

4. If I could live my life over I would choose:

5. In five years I would like to be:

6. In ten years I would like to be:

7. After all is said and done I am a dentist/dental professional because:

Now write a *Professional Mission Statement* that summarizes the essence of why you are a dentist or dental professional. Use as much space as needed.

Chapter 4

THE PRACTICE PHILOSOPHY

"I barely make it through each day. Not only do I *hate* the problems I face with my staff, but I *hate* the pressure I'm under all day long. I *hate* the fact that I can't seem to find the time to really think about my cases. I know I'm missing lots of opportunities to do more and better work for people, but I'm pulled in too many directions at once. If only I could just focus on my patients and not have to do all the rest of this *crap*!" he exclaimed, waving his hand over the mounds of paper on his desk.

"I'm never done. I tried to take it home for a while, but it just piled up there, and my wife got upset about the stacks next to the bed. I'm at least a year behind in my journals, and I sometimes don't even bother to return telephone calls. Now they tell me I'm going to have to learn to use the Internet and answer e-mail every day. I'll go out of my mind! And soon we'll all be working for some insurance company. Yesterday I had to begin a major crown and bridge treatment for a patient that I had treatment planned over two years ago. I guess the patient came in a few times for prophies, but I didn't know she was ready to start the major treatment. I didn't even remember the patient that well. Since her last visit I've taken some courses on cosmetic dentistry and others on occlusion so I wasn't even sure if I was doing the right thing for the patient."

I watched as Steve began to restack the same papers he had just shuffled through, and then reach below his chair to adjust the seat. The wind had come up outside, and the sun was beginning to set across the bay. A few sailboats were slicing through the gray water, sails set and full. It was a Tuesday evening in June. Steve had been at his office since 7:30 in the morning. He caught my gaze and looked at the boats on the bay.

"I really thought I'd be able to get in a quick sail every afternoon," He hesitated, "but it was totally unrealistic. Now I'm lucky to get a few hours in on the weekend. When I was swimming I weighed 162 pounds, no fat." Steve is a little over six feet tall. "Now I weigh 205, and my knees hurt when I jog."

I asked Steve what was really important to him, what made him happy.

"Well, my family, my friends, my house and sailing. I also want to take good care of my patients and not have too many hassles at the office," he said. "Don't get me wrong, I *really like* dentistry, it's just not what I hoped it would be."

I wasn't satisfied with this answer. I said, "Steve I'm getting a feel for the kinds of things that are wrong with your life, but I'm not sure how you define what is right for your practice." I waited for Steve to think about the question.

* * *

The formulation of a *Personal Mission Statement* is more challenging for some than it is for others. It is a necessary part of the process of designing *any* business. If the principal in the business has no clue as to his or her reason for life, then it will be impossible to craft a mission for the business. Without a *Practice Mission Statement,* the purpose of the businesses would be unknown or ambiguous. A business without a purpose is destined for failure for the simple reason that those within the business will have no common purpose, and will therefore tend to work at crossed purposes.

Steve's case is far from unique. He has a *sense* of why he is in this profession. He can articulate a few features that he likes about it but can state an equal number of negatives. He is optimistic about *dentistry,* but he doesn't feel he is personally participating in the best it has to offer. He feels a bit like an outsider in his own profession.

I gave Steve the tools that appear at the end of the last chapter for analyzing his situation and creating his own *Personal Mission Statement.* I met with Steve about two weeks later. He had made some progress as we shall see...

* * *

"I found the *Personal Mission Statement* to be the hardest part of the exercise," he told me. "I had to deal with some personal issues that I really have never dealt with before. I have tried to compartmentalize my life in a way that this process seemed at first to bring too much of me personally into my professional life. Then I began to realize that may be just exactly what my practice lacks—my own *personal commitment.* It really required me to clarify some things that I maybe never have before. Plus I had to crystallize it into language that I can communicate to someone else."

"You know you don't have to share that with anyone?"

"No! Now you tell me!" he laughed.

"It just needs to be clear enough that you could share it and be understood if you chose to," I said. "The idea is that most of us only *think* we have our life purpose clear in mind.

But when we try to actually articulate it, it isn't very clear at all."

"But why couldn't I just write my *Professional Mission Statement*? That was a whole lot easier," Steve asked.

"A business statement is nothing unless it comes from a true and clear personal foundation. If you wrote the business statement without knowing what you want personally, you could achieve it and remain stressed and unfulfilled in your profession. Don't you see? The two are inseparable, especially when you are in a field so personal and intense as dentistry," I replied. "The only way to achieve many of your personal goals is through your professional life. If you are not clear on what you seek personally, how can you find direction professionally?

"Do you want to share yours with me today?" I asked.

"Sure," Steve replied. "I think it's personal, but I'm not embarrassed by it or anything. In fact after all this work you *better read it!* I found out things I had never realized before: I am really appreciative of my patients' and my office staff's trust in me. After working through the questions, I returned to some of them and answered them again, perhaps more truthfully. Hey, my life isn't perfect, but it is better than most other peoples' lives I observe. And it is my patients who make it possible for me. I would get nowhere if they didn't trust me and accept *me,* as well as my professional diagnosis and treatment."

I volunteered, "I have several clients here in California who were very clear as dental students why they chose dentistry. It was because of the lifestyle they had witnessed among the dentists in their community. One is an avid golfer, another a surfer in Southern California, a third is a skier in the Tahoe area. Each shares with the others a common trait, the love of a particular sport, but none were quite good enough to go pro and make a living. You know what else they all have in common?"

"No, but I'll bet you're going to tell me!"

"They all share a visible and genuine care and compassion for their patients and demonstrate a true passion for dentistry. They have a love of the business of dentistry as well, and see it as a way to create opportunity to provide services only they can provide. They are very grateful for the opportunity of personal achievement and happiness that caring for these patients has created in their lives. They were motivated to *become* dentists for very personal reasons. Once in the profession, they realized the importance of their work and the responsibilities their decisions created in their lives. Each has begun the process of true mastery of his profession. The irony is, they have reaped far more personal rewards from their practices than most other dentists who may even be critical of their motivation. Through dentistry, they have created the balance in their lives that has led to true happiness. I don't know of a single CEO in corporate America who can say that. There are few middle managers who even like their jobs, let alone the company they work with. After a decade of 'downsizing' and 're-engineering,' there is little satisfaction left in the typical life of the American corporate worker. I'm sure you see it in your patients."

"Yes, I do. I've always felt somewhat jealous of the power and authority that a big corporate officer has, but I've never envied the 80 hour work weeks! I know I made the right decision to become a dentist. Now I want to have the decision translate into a more perfect balance in my life!"

Steve shared his work with me. Steve's ***Personal Mission Statement:***

My purpose in life is:
to find happiness and peace,
to dedicate myself to my family,

to contribute meaningfully to my community,
to become the best I can be in my profession.

I understand that to achieve my purpose I must:
live a healthy life style,
become and remain fit,
live a full and long life.

I believe I need the help of others to achieve my purpose:
a loving and forgiving God,
my wife and family,
true friends,
loyal and dedicated staff and co-workers,
appreciative patients.

"I see you worked hard to produce this," I complemented Steve.

"Yes, and I believe it is the first time in my life that I have seen things so clearly. Not that it's such a big deal. I think I always knew this, but I never really thought I had a philosophy about it. It's just that now I have it to look at. I might even change it sometime," he said.

"It really should be a living document that is subject to change. If you would have done this when you were 16 or 23, it would have been very different. Remember who you were and what you were thinking about then?"

"Don't remind me!"

"We need to be able to change it as we live and grow. In fact, it is a good way to measure and witness our own development," I said.

"I can see how it would be. And it really will help me when I set out to create my *Professional Mission Statement,*" he volunteered. "That process is so much simpler in the context of my written personal purpose."

"You realize that the *Professional Mission Statement* is used to clarify your own professional mission and as a contribution to the *Practice Mission Statement* that you will prepare together with your staff?" I asked.

"Yes, and I see the reason for doing it in advance. I need to be able to lead and articulate my mission very clearly to my staff, and then incorporate as much as possible their purposes for participating in the practice."

"The end result is a document that all of you share and agree upon. Each one having made a contribution and therefore a powerful commitment to the ideals expressed in your mission. How can you not succeed to meet your goals when you have that powerful an alignment of the staff?"

Steve and I celebrated his accomplishment and continued our discussion over scones and coffee at his favorite coffee shop down the street.

"I don't know how this can be enough, just writing a simple statement with my staff. It is very nice to know that I have expressed a mission, but I have so many real problems to overcome. I just feel like this is sort of wishful thinking," he said.

"What's on your mind?" I asked, recognizing this stage all too well. "Often the problems seem so overwhelming that learning and taking the first few steps to correct them seems insignificant or futile."

"After Nina left we were never able to book as many patients. It was as though she was responsible for most of our new patient referrals. Our days were less busy. So I signed on a few PPOs and even a couple of capitation contracts to fill my book. We got busier but the profits never improved. In fact, things are probably worse now than ever and I'm flooded with patients. Nina told me never to do this, but she wasn't around to keep me from signing up.

"And there are other problems too. I think Nina probably took a bit more than her salary out of the practice. She was such an efficient bookkeeper that I never really had an accountant. She did all my banking and payroll filing. All I did was find someone to do my personal taxes at the end of each year. I signed all the checks, so I don't know how she could get any money. My accountant, Jeff, who I hired after she left was very suspicious of the way my old books looked. He wanted to do an audit looking back a couple of years. I thought it would be too expensive. I suspect a lot but can't prove a thing. I even wonder if Lisa and Tami didn't know about this and quit for the same reason."

"You may still want to have your accountant look into all of that before the trail is too cold," I offered.

"Eileen and I have talked about it. We honestly feel it's time to move forward to something new. We can spend a lot of energy and anguish, and even if Jeff's right we won't feel any better and we'll have lost a lot of time. That's why we looked for a consultant and hired you. We're not interested in getting even, just getting a fresh start," Steve concluded. "I do want to ensure that whether it happened or not, it won't be possible again."

"And there are other similar issues. But I don't want to beat a dead horse about all the things I've done poorly. I just want to get things *moving* again," he said. "So what's the next step?"

"Work on your own *Practice Mission Statement,* and at our first staff meeting we'll get started on that process," I replied.

* * *

Over the next few weeks, Steve and his staff worked on the *Practice Mission Statement.* Here's what they came up with:

> *This is a practice dedicated to quality dental care. As a staff, we are committed to providing state-of-the-art services to our patients to help them achieve the highest level of health, comfort and esthetics. We want to know and understand our patients in order to provide personalized care. Our office will always be clean and comfortable, and our attention to infection control and sterility will be vigilant. We are excited and enthusiastic about our work, and that means we will strive to have fun and humor in our approach to patients. We will continue to be the best we can be through continuing education and team building. Our mission is to be the best and to have our patients tell the world.*

Anyone can throw together a high-sounding "mission" to use as a marketing image. This is not what we are demonstrating by sharing Steve's process. A marketing strategy can and should emerge from your *Practice Mission Statement* and is, in fact, one very important use of the document. But trying to devise a marketing image then living up to that image is backwards for a professional services company such as a dental practice. It is like building a pyramid from the top point down. The intended result is very clear on paper but the plan and procedures for getting there just won't work. The rest of the pyramid must be designed as well, then built *from the ground up.*

With a *Practice Mission Statement* many problems are much simpler to solve. The communication between the staff can be quickly brought to resolution by speaking in the terms of the mission. Conflict resolution becomes easier and the need for it less frequent. Goals are attainable when people know what the goals are and are held accountable for their role in achieving the goals.

The Practice Philosophy

The next step of business organization is the extension of the *Practice Mission Statement* into various forms of *Practice Philosophy*. *Practice philosophy* is the translation of the mission into the myriad activities that occur during the day to day operation of the practice. It controls and directs the philosophy behind daily activities from the moment the door is open and the lights are turned on, through the many interpersonal encounters with patients and staff, to the locking up at night.

Benefits of a written practice philosophy are felt throughout the practice. Let's take a look at some of the ways a practice will feel the positive effects that follow the effort of creating a written philosophy.

A *Practice Mission Statement* is the basis for most of the communication that occurs inside a dental practice on any given day. Most consultants will tell you that the problems they see in dental practices stem mainly from missed communication or lack of communication in varying degrees. Practices with a mission have a document to orient new staff members to the "culture" of the practice. It is used in training of new employees and the ongoing training of seasoned employees. As a working document, it changes somewhat in response to the changing conditions of the workplace, yet it is a consistent guide to the important professional mission of the dentist and the practice mission of dentist and staff. It is a tool to be used in specialist communication and understanding. It will solve the vast majority of specialist communication problems as we shall see in chapters to follow.

The elements of a *Practice Philosophy* are:

- A definition of clinical excellence (or a clinical standard). In other words, your own statement of your personal standard of care.

- A description of the "culture" of the office. The "practice culture" as you defined it from your mission. It may be one of small town informality, or one of gracious upscale hospitality or anything in between. But define it. Then be consistent in applying it.

- A marketing statement—A definition of patient satisfaction. I like to see the word "dazzle" used here. Patient satisfaction is no longer a matter of simply doing your procedures well. The patient perception of the entire practice, from the first phone call to the one the night after treatment must exceed his or her expectations. More about this in the Chapter 6, Establishing Communication Standards.

- Professionalism defined in the context of your practice. How professionalism is applied to your practice.

- A statement of the culture and process of patient care. What are the *processes* of patient care? How will they be achieved?

- The outcomes expected from patient care. What are the outcomes you seek for your patients? This doesn't refer to specific patients or individual treatment plans. But how does your *Mission* translate generally into patient outcomes? Is your desire to save the patient money? Do you want health and prevention? How about esthetically pleasing results?

- The intended interface between specialists and the practice (or the specialist practice and the referring doctors).

At this point, getting this on paper should be a relatively easy task. The hard work is done when you do the various components of the *Mission* statements. But it is important that this be on paper to be shared with the staff and referring doctors and specialists. In conversations with many dentists over the years it is clear that nearly all of them have some concept of their practice philosophy. Yet it is nearly impossible to get most to express any more than a simple thought. Something like "I treat everyone to the best of my ability," or "We're a 'state-of-the-art' practice," are typical responses. These do little to provide a guide for office procedures and protocols, business systems, communication and patients' care on a daily basis. In fact, many of these dentists are quite upset when a seasoned employee cannot express a philosophy that resonates with the doctor's. The doctor reacts with: "After all these years, that's all you know about '*my philosophy'?"*

The formulation and writing of a *Personal Mission Statement* and *Practice Mission Statement* is a sticking point for many dentists. Yet it is one of the elements common to most highly successful practices. I cannot emphasize its importance enough. If you had trouble with the last chapter, you are not alone. But understand that there are no shortcuts to excellence. The formulation of a *Practice Mission Statement* provides the foundation for all that comes next.

Most dentists who work through the process of creating a mission find they have some very noble and altruistic motivations among the elements that they express in their mission. This can be in contrast with the reality of their practice situation. Discovering this is not a comfortable feeling and can lead to a great deal of self-criticism and guilt. It is important to remember that the circumstances that led to whatever your current situation may be were the past events of your life and practice. They led you to where you are today without the benefit of the type of understanding and planning that you are now gaining. The circumstances of a life that bring a person to a juncture must always be considered when one is tempted to become judgmental.

Sharing the process of the *Practice Mission Statement* with your staff begins the process of putting your house in order. The foundation has been established with the participation of those best able to assist you in achieving your practice goals. Writing a *Practice Philosophy* translates these concepts into a communication tool to help you run the practice effectively.

Now it is time to translate the *Practice Philosophy* into practical, working systems that define, describe and implement your practice philosophy. It will include the policies and procedures you employ to apply that philosophy to the care of your patients and the operation of your business. "Oh no! Not more writing," you say. Yes, and let me explain...

The world we live in today is ever more complex. Where procedures were once simple and routine, now they are high tech. Where margins were once an unmeasured thickness of zinc phosphate cement, now they are delicate and seamless bonded materials measured in microns. Where success in practice was once a simple matter of telling one or two employees how you wanted something to be done, today there are hundreds of critical tasks.

But what is really important is not always what seems the most obvious. The tasks are not an end in themselves, but the result of a set of business systems that allow the tasks to occur. It just seems that the tasks are an entire function of the office. The organizations that we create in society, including dental practices, are what implement the business performance. It is no longer a solo effort, but the effort of the combined *behaviors* of numerous people in an organization. The formal structure of the organization and its ability to be managed are what hold successful businesses (and dental practices) together. Informal organizations are seductive. It just seems that it is so much easier if we can keep things on an "informal" level, sort of like a family. Yet look at how the family is being shattered in today's society; fewer than 50 percent of all children will be raised by two parents by the year 2000. Perhaps more formal organizational structure should be applied to families.

Defining the purpose of the practice and translating that into a working philosophy is the actual substance of the organization. It is the means to an end. And that end is the business performance and the results obtained by that performance. To do less, even in the smallest practice is to doom it to failure, a failure likely to come soon because of the rapid changes in the business environment.

So the *Practice Philosophy* needs to be written and reviewed often. It need not be a lengthy manifesto but simply a statement which brings the *Practice Mission Statement* into workable terms. This allows the mission to be grafted into every policy and procedure that is followed in the organization.

Chapter 5

COMMUNICATING YOUR PHILOSOPHY

Steve's situation is far from unique. It is common among dentists in every community around the country, whether or not managed care's impact has yet been felt. Dentists are experiencing a change in the manner in which dental practice is conducted. The old rules no longer apply, and many of the new ones have proven faint help. The loss of control over the individual dentist's practice, whether from the intrusion of managed care, or other market forces, has resulted in a loss of clinical quality standards and the increase in risks being assumed by the individual dentist. Such risks are both the financial risks of a less forgiving market environment, and the liability risks of reduced clinical standards coupled with increasing patient expectations. Not a pretty picture from the standpoint of professional malpractice risk!

But, more importantly, the frustration level of dentists with their professional lives is rising fast. The reason for the lack of control isn't always definable. Dentists often differ in where they place the cause or the blame. The answers from managers and advisers have not come at the same pace, nor have they been accurate and effective. So dentists are worried, and for good reason. We take a look at our colleagues in medicine and wonder, "Are we really as different as the gurus claim? Or will dentistry be the next profession to be absorbed by the new American Insurance Economy?"

"Remember that patient I told you I was unhappy about starting a treatment the last time we met?" Steve asked next.

"The one you weren't sure if you should begin?" I replied.

"Yes, that one. She reminded me of another case. It's kind of an illustration of many of my frustrations with this practice."

"Tell me about her," I invited.

"Mary Ann did not have a particularly memorable new patient exam," Steve began. "I remember talking to her on the first visit and recommending quite a large treatment plan. We did the usual exam, bitewings and a Pano and all."

"How long did it take?" I asked.

"Oh, my exams take about 15 minutes, sometimes a bit more. Depends on whether I do a perio chart or leave it to the hygienist."

"How often is that?" I asked.

"Well, usually I defer the exam and review the measurements later. That day, though, the patient slipped through the cracks. She never got a perio exam," Steve confessed. "So when she came in several months later, scheduled for all six anteriors to be crowned, I went ahead with the treatment. We completed that, plus the upper posteriors, and a lower quadrant of bridge work within the next 18 months or so. She seemed happy with the work and it looked really good.

"What I didn't realize was she *never* saw my hygienist, and though her X-rays were pretty unremarkable, she had some pretty significant pocketing here and there. Now, don't get me wrong, this is *not* my standard of care, but somehow Mary Ann slipped between the stools. I really laid into my staff for that one when I found out. They *know* how I want my patients handled.

"Anyway, when she had the crowns on the anteriors for about six months and the gums were still inflamed, she complained to my receptionist, who scheduled an appointment with my hygienist, Liz. When Liz saw her, she probed, and was quite alarmed. She called me into the room. I confirmed that there was pretty significant periodontal disease and the pockets would need treatment. We did everything right from that point, informed the patient, began non-surgical soft tissue management, and home care instructions, but things just went from bad to worse.

"We decided to refer Mary Ann to my periodontist, Dr. Joe Larson. Joe is a great guy and a really good periodontist, but I think he blew it in Mary Ann's case."

"Why do you say that?" I asked.

"He sent me a note describing her condition, which was no surprise, then outlined a surgical treatment plan. I figured he'd be careful, knowing the crowns were new and all, but the result was horrible. There were exposed margins and black triangles all across the front, and Mary Ann was furious! She called me on the telephone, refused to come back here, even to let me redo the crowns for free. She said Dr. Larson told her the crowns should not have been done prior to the surgery, and she took that to mean I am incompetent. She would not tell me where she was going next, but later she filed a complaint with my local peer review committee. I found out she had been to a prosthodontist group across the bay. She told the peer review that she needed all of her work remade.

"I went to peer review. They found that my exam was incomplete, but my treatment was within the standard of care since I did eventually address her periodontal needs. They recommended she allow me to remake the crowns, but she refused. She then hired an attorney and they were going to sue me, so my malpractice carrier settled with her for the cost of the remakes in the other office. I think we got off pretty lucky, but none of it would have happened if my staff and Dr. Larson had followed my protocols," he complained.

"How do they know your protocols?" I asked.

"I talk about my standards and procedures *all the time,*" Steve answered. "They should know from being around me that I have high integrity and want only the best for my patients! Plus they can observe what I do, and if they'd only follow my directions...."

"Whoa!" I interrupted. "Let's back up and talk about how your staff and referred specialists are supposed to *understand* your standards of care if you haven't ever written them down. I think that's expecting an awful lot, don't you? They aren't the ones ultimately responsible for the result, are they?"

"Well, no," Steve hesitated, "but they are responsible for following my directions and delivering the services I expect!"

"Procedures you expect or procedures you actually communicate?" I asked.

"I see your point," he said. "They can only do what I've *actually* communicated needs to be done specifically for each individual patient. But in a busy practice, that's *impossible*!" he protested. "So much of what we do is absolutely routine, and the doctor shouldn't have to order every patient napkin and cotton roll!" He was almost shouting now, annoyed by the apparent absurdity of what I was asking.

"Steve, my point is not that you have to order every two by two." I offered, mirroring his sarcasm. "Only that it has to be ordered *somehow, and somewhere,* either by verbal command or direction or by written standing orders or standard operating procedures."

"So now we need a book of procedures?" he asked.

"Only for those things you want to avoid doing wrong or forgetting, or getting sued over," I answered.

Steve looked out over the bay. The sails of the boats were fiery gold in the light of the setting sun, and the wind was beginning to calm.

Getting Your Ideas on Paper

The staff knows you and your philosophy, right? So do all your specialists, correct?

Don't bet on it. The staff probably loves you and respects you, but they are not dentists. They do not have your education, background or understanding of the complex problems you solve. They have no clue what kinds of pressures you are under to run the business and take care of the patients. And they are human beings with all the wonderful frailties we share. Imagine that one day you have clinical care on your mind, and deliver a lengthy and detailed lesson on the importance of some details of clinical procedures. The next day you are feeling pressure because of a growing receivables situation and past due bills, and you react to that. A few days later, when everyone is on the phone trying to reduce the A/R and your procedure is stalled because of a poor clinical tray set-up, you erupt with anger or seethe with cynicism. Why? Because you are sending a variety of mixed and incompatible signals about your philosophy to your staff. They react in ways that are predictable, human and understandable. Yet their result is an unhappy doctor.

Sound familiar? If your answer is no, then go *ask your staff.* I'll bet you get a different answer. Or they may be afraid to answer honestly. And that is just one example. I have visited literally dozens of dental offices and have taught or consulted hundreds of dentists. One thing I find very common is this: *Dentists are not very clear in their communications.* They are busy. Communication in dental offices tends to be incomplete and ambiguous when observed over time. More disturbing is the fact that patients are present to witness a lot of missed communication, passive aggressive behavior and cynicism and even overt anger. Is this any way to run a business?

Dr. Rich Green of the L.D. Pankey Institute shared a metaphor for this condition with me. He describes the dentist as a juggler. There is really no foundation upon which we can base our operations that is as solid as the little diagrams that we draw. I really like pyramid diagrams and have several to illustrate such things as the principles of practice management or the principles of personal finance. But this is not what happens in truth. Each little area of our life is not so easily sequestered, though we need to do so to learn and understand how things work and how to manage them.

So we are like jugglers. Then what happens is we always have too many balls in the air. Life is fine when the balls are all up there, balanced in a nice trajectory through space and time. But when one falls down into our hand, we must deal with it. It may be the *Financial Arrangements Ball,* or the *Personnel Communications Ball,* or perhaps the *Clinical Procedures Ball.* If we have done our job well, the ball that falls does so in proper time and concert with the other balls and we can deal with it. We toss it up in the air where it is fine once again. Then another one comes down. It may be the *Accounts Receivables Ball* or the *Equipment Acquisition and Financing Ball.* And this goes on for the life of the practice. As long as we are balanced and concentrate on all the balls, but pay special attention to the ones falling into our hands, everything works out. Right? The problems emerge when we lose our balance or concentration. Then there are balls falling all around, pounding us on the head, bouncing off the floor and walls, rolling under foot. Chaos. And stress.

The solution is to have a written *Practice Philosophy* so that at any time many of the balls live happily in a display case and you never have to juggle all of them at once. You have control of the practice and *choose* which balls to select for juggling at any point in time. The *Practice Philosophy* is a document that allows you to communicate continuously with every member of your staff and to deal with them from a position of mutual understanding.

Your philosophy becomes a way to translate your mission statements into reality. It is then a tool to communicate how the practice will operate with regard to the staff, the patients, and the various other practices—either specialists or referring doctors. You must communicate successfully to attain your goals. Imagine that every time you begin a staff meeting or a personnel conference or employee evaluation you have in your arms a small, bound book or ring binder that tells you and your staff the philosophy that guides every decision you are about to make.

The benefits to you and you staff are clear communications and smooth daily operations. Like employees in any effective organization, dental staff persons need guidance. It can come from many sources. The best one is from the doctor but this is impractical if he or she is to be productive in the clinical area. As doctors we simply cannot spend our time directing and guiding all the systems implemented by staff individually each day. The *Practice Philosophy* is a guide that comes from the doctor to the staff, providing a daily resource to explain, enhance and coordinate the concepts of staff functions.

Patients benefit as well. A new patient first arriving to the office will be greeted in a manner consistent with how she was treated during her initial telephone interview. If she was treated with deferential respect, she will feel that as she walks into the reception room for the first time. If she was initially treated with a warm, friendly and casual approach, the receptionist will convey that feeling. It is a matter of philosophy of how you wish your patients to be approached. Done correctly it will help attract the kind of patients you want to your practice. Whether you are the deferential type, or the warm and casual type, or even the happy-go-lucky or the professorial, you can apply your leadership skills your way. Use of a written practice philosophy allows you to lead in your own style, and attract to your practice those patients most likely to respond to your personality and demeanor. None of us can be all things to all people. We fail terribly when we try. It is better to present a chosen office personality and culture, develop it, and be consistent in its implementation by applying your *Practice Philosophy.*

Perhaps the greatest benefit comes to all the stakeholders in the practice—the doctor, staff, patients and *referring doctors or specialists*—by the use of the *Practice Philosophy* in specialist communications. Specialist and referring doctor communications often lead to less than satisfactory results. In fact, in many office protocols there is no direct communication between the doctors at all regarding a particular referred patient. This can lead to a liability disaster in cases where clinical expectations are not met. It often goes something like this:

* * *

Steve had been working on applying his *Practice Philosophy* for a few days. We were talking prior to a staff meeting to discuss some difficulties he had experienced with his oral surgeon.

"My assistant, Kim, made the call since Dena was busy at the desk," he said. "We had a patient in the chair who had an infection, a pericoronitis with facial swelling getting worse in the lower right side. I used to do a lot of surgery but got away from it when my practice was busy. When I took on the CAP and PPO plans I started getting stung financially for referring surgery to specialists, so I started doing my own surgeries again. But this one was complicated. There was a lot of swelling, the patient had some medical problems, and I had just had some bad post-operative problems from another similar case. So I decided to refer."

"Do you have a good relationship with the surgeon?" I asked.

"Well, there's where the problem started. I really don't have a good working relationship with a particular surgeon since I do so much of my own surgery," he said. "So I had Kim call this one I used a few times. There is one that I liked better, but I burned that bridge, or at least I thought I did when I stopped referring patients to him. Over the years I've used several different surgeons. It seems they're really attentive at first. Then they stop being as concerned or interested toward me or my patients. One, Dr. Grimes, was even quite arrogant and demeaning to some of my patients."

"There's certainly no shortage of available surgeons to choose from in this area," I said.

"I know," Steve replied, "and I think I've tried them all. For some reason it just doesn't work out over the long haul.

"Anyway, Kim called the office and talked to the surgeon's receptionist. She said they could not see the patient until the next morning. In the meantime, we should give him antibiotics. Kim knows my usual regimen, so she first checked the patient's chart for allergies or previous medical problems and then wrote a prescription for me to sign."

"I think I know where this is leading," I said.

"You can't even imagine how bad this got," Steve said. "The patient got rapidly worse. He never called me or my surgeon. He just went to the hospital that night and was treated by the emergency room physicians with I.V. antibiotics, and they did some sort of external incision and drainage. They kept him there overnight and referred him to a different oral surgeon the next day. It happens to be the arrogant one, Dr. Grimes, with whom I had problems before. Well, bad went to worse and this guy calls me to tell me I failed to observe the proper standards of surgical care, and he had half a mind to report me to the State Board. Plus, he would not listen to the fact that I had acted according to the recommendations from another oral surgeon.

"By this time I was sweating. I called the oral surgeon I had referred the patient to, and he said he had not been informed of any patient from my office. He did not make any recommendations, and he always sees emergencies on the same day."

I interrupted: "So you had one dental assistant school graduate talking to probably a high school graduate on the phone, solving clinical problems that the doctors didn't have time for, and the patient winds up in the hospital."

"That's about it," Steve confessed. "You can see how quickly the situation deteriorated without *either* the surgeon or me even knowing what was happening. Fortunately, Grimes didn't follow through on his threat."

"Probably because he had second thoughts about a specialist turning in his referring doctor on a situation that wasn't clearly substandard," I suggested.

"Right. The guy has lost a lot of business because of his attitude," Steve said. "He really is a great technical surgeon. He just has a terrible professional manner.

"So can I prevent this from ever happening again? Obviously I will be more diligent about getting on the phone when situations are unusual. But I don't think I need to discuss every case with my specialists, do I?"

"I think it is an excellent policy to have a clinical conference by telephone on every case," I answered. "But it isn't always possible to coordinate the two doctors with a telephone conference when each one is busy with clinical procedures on patients. The demands of clinical dentistry, coupled with the dangers of contamination and the protocols for infection control make it nearly impossible to interrupt most procedures to take a call. It becomes even less possible in a surgeon's or periodontist's practice."

"So what do we do?" Steve asked.

We learn by repetition, so I am never apologetic for repeating a concept or idea. "We begin by returning to your practice mission," I said. "There we will find that you are 'dedicated to quality care,' that you 'know and understand your patients,' and that your patients will achieve the 'highest level of health comfort and esthetics.' Seems you fell a bit short in that case."

"Did we ever."

"But remember, the *Practice Mission* didn't exist at the time, so you and your staff had a different set of rules you were laboring under. Now to prevent this from happening, and to improve your patients' outcomes, we need to translate the mission into a philosophy that helps to implement the mission."

"Do I then share this with my specialists?" Steve asked.

"More than that, you will find you want to have a mutual statement of philosophy that defines and guides the culture, process and expectations of the outcomes for patients of the two practices." I offered. "That way, it isn't a directive from you that your specialist must bend to comply with, but a statement of mutual obligations and agreements that will benefit the individual patient and each practice. You can imagine the reception such a document might get from the oral surgeon who wanted to report you. Yet he could become your best ally in practice if you could establish a mutual understanding of each of your expectations."

"So I kind of 'enroll' the specialists in my philosophy?" he laughed.

"Exactly. One at a time, specific to their practice. And limit the number of specialists you refer to so you aren't overwhelmed by this process. Each one of them will have a lot to say about how *they* see patient care, much of which you will likely agree with. Then *you* take the task of putting it in a written statement. By taking the lead, it will look much like your own philosophy statement but will also reflect the input from the particular specialist." I said.

"Each specialist will then have in possession a ***Joint Statement of Philosophy*** that will guide the journey each patient has through the referral process and the clinical care they receive. Once the *Joint Statement of Philosophy* is completed, you could never have a situation develop like the ones you described. They would simply fall too far from the implemented philosophy—lots of alarms would be going off in both practices. Of course for that to happen, the philosophy must be translated into training for each staff."

"And you want me to believe that most dentists have implemented a project like this?" he asked in disbelief.

"No—only the most successful ones—the dentists who are fulfilling their dreams," I replied.

Steve's Sample Specialist Joint Statement of Philosophy:

Our practice exists to provide the highest quality restorative and preventive dental care in a relationship-based practice, with a highly qualified staff of caring professionals, in a comfortable and pleasant environment, to patients who appreciate our efforts and commitment to this level of care.

To that end, we need to establish and promote open and continuous clinical communication regarding our standards of care, methods, procedures, patient progress and outcomes.

This is a general practice which emphasizes comprehensive quality restorative care. We are dedicated to achieving the goals of patient comfort, function, esthetics and long-term stability of the stomatognathic system for our patients. In order to achieve such a complete result, predictably and efficiently, we have certain standards of clinical practice that we demand of ourselves, and expect from our participating specialists. These standards are incorporated into our general methods of patient management.

New Patient Exam

The new patient exam is not a single event but a process that may involve several visits over a period of time from a few days to many months, or in certain cases, even years.

1. Evaluation and initial treatment of emergency or other compelling problems.
2. Pre-clinical interview: This is for behavioral and motivational assessment of the patient and gives us a chance to meet and understand the patient's needs and desires. We classify the patient according to personality type and dental I.Q. We will share our evaluations and operating conclusions with our specialists in our introductory letters.
3. Clinical Examination: An interactive evaluation using theories of "co-diagnosis" to involve the patient in the discovery and planning processes.

   a. Medical and Dental History
   b. Intraoral Imaging
   c. Intraoral examination of the dentition, periodontal structures, soft tissues of the oral-pharynx and pharynx and an evaluation of the dental occlusion.
   d. Head and neck examination of surface structures, muscles, skin, TM joints.
4. All findings are recorded in our standard format, using written documentation.
5. Complete appropriate radiographs and imaging.
6. Diagnostic study models. These are mounted in any case of occlusal disease, TMD or in cases of anticipated restorative treatment planning.
7. Referrals will be made during the diagnostic stages to associated specialty practitioners from our select list.
8. Final treatment planning is conducted after all fact finding has been completed.
9. Clinical planning conferences are held as necessary with specialists in order to plan and coordinate complex treatment.

Clinical Consultation

This is a meeting in my consultation room and includes the patient, a staff member who takes notes of the meeting, and in rare cases, one or more specialists.

1. Communicate the findings from the comprehensive patient evaluation including a summary of specialists' findings.
2. Diagnosis of all conditions. Report to the patient any pathology including tooth wear, mobility, periodontal conditions, TM joint conditions, soft tissue conditions, serviceability of current restorations, causes of breakdown of dentition, etc.

3. An initial treatment plan is presented. This should include a prediction of the anticipated final treatment plan to give the patient a clear idea of the general scope of expected treatment.
4. Later, additional consultations are conducted with the patient as results of initial therapies such as occlusal therapy and initial periodontal therapy are evaluated. Further treatment plans are formulated and presented.
5. Comprehensive treatment plans are presented after the results of initial therapy including periodontal therapy, occlusal therapy and trial equilibration on mounted study models.

Occlusal Splint Therapy

This practice emphasizes harmony and balance of the entire occlusal-muscle-TMJ system. Definitive restorative therapy is completed in centric relation occlusion or in cases of degenerative joint disease or TMD, in a stable adapted centric position or posture. The need for occlusal therapy is evaluated during the initial patient examination and thereafter during initial therapy. The doctor may determine the need for occlusal splint therapy during these early stages of the new patient process, or such needs may emerge at various times in the course of caring for a patient in the practice.

1. Initial determination is made of the need for occlusal splint therapy.
2. Indications include but are not limited to:
   a. Symptoms of TMD
   b. Symptoms of occlusal-muscle disharmony
   c. Tooth wear indicated by facets, abfractions, loss of enamel, chipping, cracking, rough surfaces
   d. Mobility of teeth
   e. Periodontal disease

   f. Any masticatory disfunction that is caused by a disorder of the occlusal-muscle relationship
3. Goals of treatment: To evaluate the effects on the TM joint and occlusal-muscle system by creating idealized occlusal function upon the splint.
   a. Anterior guidance
   b. Immediate posterior disclusion upon excursions
   c. Bilateral, maximal number of equal intensity posterior occlusal stops in centric relation, adapted centric posture, or treatment posture subject to evaluation

Definitive Occlusal Therapy

Definitive occlusal therapy may include equilibration, comprehensive restorative dentistry, orthodontics, or oral surgery to achieve the result of a stable centric relation occlusion or adapted centric posture for our patient.

1. Mounted study models are evaluated.
2. Desired treatment outcomes are designed and completed by modification of the stone models. This may include:
   a. Trial equilibration
   b. Tooth model modification to imitate predicted or desired results from orthodontic therapy
   c. Alveolar model modification to simulate predicted or desired results from alveolar or orthognathic surgery
3. Modifications are preserved by duplicating the waxed model modifications with reversible hydrocolloid and a new stone model.
4. When an acceptable occlusal relationship can be achieved on the models by trial equilibration, and it is anticipated that correction of the occlusal disharmony

will correct the masticatory disfunction, equilibration is completed on the patient.

5. When an acceptable result is not possible with a combination of equilibration and restorative treatment, the patient is referred for appropriate orthodontic evaluation.
6. Most completed cases require long term protection of the stomatognathic system with protective or physiologic occlusal splinting, usually at night only.

Specialist Relations

A patient may at any time have the need for evaluation and care by one or more dental specialty practitioners. Our specialty referrals are made only to a select group of qualified doctors who have made a shared commitment to our practice philosophy and have a similar and mutually inclusive practice philosophy.

Patients must not become subjected to confusion or controversy over clinical philosophy, behavioral approaches, management styles, financial arrangements, diagnosis or treatment planning over the course of their experience in and between our offices. Clinical disagreements or differences of opinion must be first discussed by the doctors and agreement reached so patients are not exposed to unnecessary ambiguity due to their interaction with several practitioners. In the case of equally viable clinical alternatives, the doctors should come to an agreement on a ordered list of differential diagnoses, and prioritized treatment recommendations before presenting case conclusions to the patient. When definitive diagnosis or treatment planning is not possible because of the need for evaluative procedures, such as initial periodontal therapy or occlusal splint therapy, the doctors should discuss the case in sufficient detail to be able to communicate the initial diagnosis and treatment plan with the patient in similar, consistent terms, and with clarity.

1. Referrals may emanate from either this practice or a specialty practice. Mutuality of patient referral is an expected practice.
2. Upon referral, the referring doctor will provide a letter of patient introduction including:
   a. Patient vital statistics
   b. Initial examination results
   c. Behavioral and motivational evaluations
   d. Reasons for the referral
   e. Request for examination and/or therapy
3. The doctor who receives the referral will conduct an examination.
4. Thereafter, the treating doctors (two or more) will hold a clinical conference either in person or by teleconference to discuss clinical findings and plan initial or comprehensive treatment.
5. Initial specialty treatments are incorporated into the comprehensive treatment plan.
6. I will summarize the results of all the specialist diagnosis and treatment planning during my initial case consultation with the patient.
7. Each specialist will conduct his or her own detailed treatment consultations with the patient and obtain appropriate consent for those specific treatments.
8. Clinical consultations between the doctors will be held by telephone periodically during the course of therapy in the specialty practice.
9. Treatment completion and final outcomes, plus plans for continued care or follow-up will be communicated by letter from the treating specialist.

Staff Enrollment

This style of practice cannot be maintained without the complete commitment and enrollment of a quality staff. They must be team players who understand and promote among each other the qualities and benefits of exceptional team performance. The following is a standard operating procedure that I use to hire and evaluate top team members.

TEAMWORK EVALUATION

[teameval.5]

Desired Outcome: Develop individuals who work exceptionally well together as a team to maximize overall performance of the staff in meeting or exceeding our goals.

Measurement: Give a score of U=0, NA=1, S=2, VG=3, E=4 for each criterion, then average the score. Each staff member must score a 2.5 or better or make remedial efforts to demonstrate improvement. All scores below 3.5 must have an action plan for improvement. Our goal is a staff of "4's"!

Method: Each quarter complete the following assessment tool for each employee. This may be more often than the employee performance evaluation. Offer assistance in helping the staff person develop and monitor an action plan for improvement.

TEAMWORK EVALUATION

Name ______________________________ Date ________
Position ______________________ Date of Hire ________
Evaluator ____
Current Performance Rating _______
Previous Overall Performance Rating _______

Description of General Behavioral Criteria
for all Staff Members

- Insuring the safety and well-being of patients
- Serving as a role model for other staff

Teamwork Evaluation \ 2

- Assisting the doctor in achieving the goals of the practice
- Solving interpersonal problems without intervention
- Providing teamwork and commitment to others
- Enforcing policies and procedures or suggesting positive ways to change

Specific Considerations:

Responsibility

E Very responsible; sets an example for others; patients are #1 concern

VG Sets a good example for staff; above average effort

S Sets a fair example; does enough to do the job well

NA Weak in responsibility; does not take any leadership roles

U Irresponsible; sets a poor example; acts immature or condescending

Area Management

E Always in control of area of work responsibility; uses positive techniques for work group interactions; maintains a safe and happy atmosphere in the office

Teamwork Evaluation \ 3

VG Always in the work area; generally positive with co-workers

S Some difficulty getting the tasks completed; some time spent in unproductive or unrelated tasks

NA Inattention to details; unable to get the job done; doctor and others must frequently fill in or answer simple questions

U Poor judgment; negative with co-workers and patients

Cooperation

E Great team worker, accepts and seeks the help of others; works towards the goals of the practice; patient care is first

VG Good teamworker; generally looks out for others; accepts direction

S Fair teamworker; somewhat self-centered or unresponsive to other's needs on occasion; could be more productive if more attentive and receptive to others

NA Difficulty working with others; self-centered; difficulty maintaining a safe, productive and happy environment

Teamwork Evaluation \ 4

U Self-centered; negative toward the practice and the other team members; does not support the practice goals

Enthusiasm

E Contagious, enthusiastic involvement; usually upbeat and enthusiastic, even for unpleasant tasks; never complains or brings others down

VG Good involvement and participation; generally enthusiastic about most activities and duties

S Mentally engaged; not overtly enthusiastic, but never negative

NA Has difficulty even promoting an enthusiastic atmosphere; mocks others' enthusiasm

U Cynical or sarcastic in relating to others; negative involvement with activities in practice: "Another prep?" or "Why do ***I*** always get that job?"

Problem Solving

E Determines the problems that can be solved alone and does so; decides which need group interaction or action plans or need adjustment of goals—then positively presents the problem to others

Teamwork Evaluation \ 5

VG Recognizes most problems; deals with most of them alone; shares well with staff

S Recognizes some problems and attempts solutions; takes too many to the doctor or other staff because of inability or unwillingness to attempt solutions alone

NA Difficulty discerning problems; tries to hand everything off to another person; very literal with job description; avoids unpleasant problems

U Compounds problems; promotes difficulty, even seems to like to observe failure by someone else or the team; "I told you so!" personality

<u>Conformity with mission, goals, policies and procedures</u>

E Is enthusiastically supportive of the office mission and goals; gets behind every policy or makes positive efforts to modify; always conforms to established procedures, but again is creative and proactive about changing things that don't work

VG Quietly supportive of mission and goals; gets in and does the job according to the policies and procedures; does not need to be reminded to conform

Teamwork Evaluation \ 6

S Gets the job done with few reminders or discussion; does not complain about procedures or policies; is not passionate about the mission but never negative either

NA Lax about procedures; ignores policies except when confronted; does not really understand the mission

U Ignores the procedures and policies; negative or disbelieving of the mission; needs to be asked or reminded to conform to office culture

Effort

E Constantly making a contribution; conscientious and careful; high level of initiative—a true self-starter; finds the work; gets more done in a day than is really expected

VG Works hard; helps out wherever needed; looks for tasks and opportunities to help; takes others lead before jumping to it

S Gets the job done without constant supervision; needs some daily guidance as to tasks; does not "see" work needed to be done; no complaints, though, and prefers to be busy, just needs help in getting lists of tasks, etc.

Teamwork Evaluation \ 7

NA Needs lots of supervision; hesitant to get on with the job, a foot dragger; comfortable leaving incomplete tasks—even for others; needs to asked to help when others are clearly busy

U Poor effort; needs to be asked and continuously supervised; complains or passively resists when asked to join in or help; feels like he/she is doing more than others and not being recognized; unaware of effort put forth by others

OVERALL PERFORMANCE:

Assign numbers to each score. Add the scores and divide by seven. This will be the "Performance Rating." Enter the number below and at the top of the evaluation for easy reference. Assign a verbal score: i.e., "Very Good."

TOTAL SCORE: ______ (÷ 7) = __________

EXCELLENT ___

VERY GOOD ___

SATISFACTORY ___

NEEDS ATTENTION* ___

UNEMPLOYED ___

Teamwork Evaluation \ 8

*This used to be "Needs Improvement," but in today's less forgiving economic environment there is insufficient time to council and train people with this rating. They must have some very high ratings in certain areas to create a belief in their potential to be an excellent employee.

Note: All employees are expected to be moving toward the "Excellent" rating in their job performance. An employee with only a satisfactory rating is not a great employee. A single "U" rating is essentially a cause for firing. Just document everything.

ACTION PLAN FOR IMPROVEMENT

[actionpl.5]

1. Score the evaluation. Give an overall result.
2. Select any criterion which is 2 or below and include in action plan.
3. If no criterion is below 2, select the lowest three for action.
4. If the employee is an exceptional employee, select areas where the employee feels he or she is anxious to improve in some way. Do not accept complacency or believe someone with all 4's needs no further improvement. All humans can improve continuously throughout life.
5. Set up a three month action plan:

AREA(S) OF FOCUS

____

____

____

____

____

____

____

IMPROVEMENT PLAN

____

____

____

____

____

____

____

Action Plan For Improvement / 2

ACTION TAKEN

____

____

____

____

____

____

BY DATE ____________

REVIEW BY (Name) ___________________________

Chapter 6

ESTABLISHING COMMUNICATION STANDARDS

"I'm afraid I'll lose them if I overwhelm them with such a detailed treatment plan!" Steve worried out loud. "Most of my patients only want to do the minimum, and they all seem to be limited in their finances to what their insurance will pay."

"I hear that from nearly every dentist I talk with." I replied. "Yet I can assure you the really successful doctors present and achieve very high patient acceptance of extensive, comprehensive treatment plans."

"I just don't see how. I am not that confident, and I'm really afraid that the patient will object and reject my treatment plan. Where will I go then?" Steve asked.

"You can hide in the lab." I joked.

"Yeah, that's about what it feels like. But seriously, how do they do it? I mean, the doctors who get this kind of acceptance?" He asked.

"There is no simple answer to that question" I began. "The elements of successful case presentation are sincerity, preparation, simplicity, clarity and persuasion. If any of those are missing, you will have difficulty with case acceptance."

"So it's not just a matter of some simple 'sales formula' like I hear about from other management consultants?" he probed.

"No, because the most important ingredient is sincerity," I replied, "and you can't fake that with some sales pitch. The way to become confident and assured during a case presentation is to be sincere, to keep the patient's needs first and foremost in your mind, to imagine the successful outcome at the end of treatment and to be yourself. Professionalism has nothing to do with being aloof or unapproachable. The patients will accept treatment from a doctor they feel knows them, is sincere and therefore trustworthy, and is open to revealing himself to the patients."

"It's a two way relationship." Steve offered.

Essentials of Communication

If there is a single word or concept that best describes the problems encountered in less effective practices, and is the defining difference found in the top echelon of effective dental practice, it is *communication*. Communication defines and creates the mood, image and environment of a practice. It establishes the basis for relationships with patients, between the doctor and the staff, and among the staff, as well as those important relationships with specialists or referring doctors. Communication provides the means for completion of important tasks and functions from the image projected by the person answering the first telephone call from a prospective patient, to the lab slip with a cryptic "PFM #14—A-2" sent to a lab in another state.

Communication will make or break your practice. Too often it is taken for granted.

The lack of effective communication influences every task and event in the practice. Staff members without clear job criteria and feedback on performance are far less effective than those with excellent job descriptions and regular performance reviews. Crowns that do not have the beauty, color, contour, and occlusion that the doctor "expects" from his lab are often not due to a poorly trained or incapable technician, but are a result of communication problems. Patients who complain about the discourteous or impersonal service they received from "your" oral surgeon's staff are a symptom of poor communication between the two offices, as well as with the patients. Even a poor periodontal surgical result can be partly explained by incomplete or misdirected communication. And the doctor's greatest fear—a malpractice lawsuit—is almost *always* from poor communications with your patient. People who understand and like each other simply do not sue each other.

THE PURPOSE OF COMMUNICATION

Patient Outcomes

Stated the most simply, the purpose of all dental practice communication is to create *positive patient outcomes.* Everything else stems from the positive outcomes experienced by the patients in the practice. When patient after patient experiences their perceived dental needs being met, with great value added in the forms of hospitality, personal relationships, understanding, and clinical competence, the practice will succeed. We often feel that we know what is best for the patient and strive to provide such services. But in absence of communication, the most exquisite dentistry will simply not be appreciated by any but the most knowledgeable and discerning patient. It would be nice to find that great dentistry would create a practice filled with such patients, but that is not the case. Your patients have no basis to evaluate the quality of your work, so without clear and effective communication that demonstrates the difference between mediocrity and clinical excellence, the patients do not know the excellence they have experienced. They have nothing to tell their friends.

The benefits to the patient in personal health, beautiful appearance, freedom from discomfort and all the other positive features of modern dentistry completed with exquisite results should be the primary motivation of any dental practice. The secondary effects of those patient services are the prosperity of the practice and therefore the doctor and his or her staff, practice growth through positive word of mouth marketing and the intrinsic rewards of being in such a great profession.

The Heart of Communication

Keeping the patient at the heart of all communication is one way to maintain this important ordering of priorities. Looking first to marketing and revenue effects is a mistake, since the efforts will be seen as shallow and self-serving by discerning patients.

Communication takes many forms. We all understand that the things we say are communication. But are they really? If the listener heard something different than the speaker thought he or she said, communication has not occurred; at least not accurate communication because each person leaves the conversation with a different thought or result in mind.

Communication can occur through direct interpersonal contact including the telephone and written messages or through other non-personal media communication such as e-mail or audio or video recordings. It may also come second hand. In some large offices communication is often more remote than "second hand," and may be removed from the originator by three or four people. It is no surprise that the result is completely different than the originator expected.

Direct, oral personal communication is not always clear. It is influenced by:

- spoken words
- verbal cues in tone and emphasis
- body language
- eye contact
- pace, whether rushed or not rushed
- attitude of the speaker, whether patronizing or overly deferential
- attitude of the listener, including nervousness or anxiety

Written and other media communications are often clearer. They are less influenced by the variables listed above, and can be referred to any number of times for clarity and consistency. Electronic media communication includes other media such as audio and video recordings, broadcast media and e-mail. The flood of new ways that we are now processing and conveying information has caused an overload for many people. You might say it has complicated the process, muddied the waters somewhat, and made us less able to communicate clearly and from the heart. So our task is as important as ever, and perhaps more difficult than ever.

Patient Response is the Communication

In our efforts to achieve patient understanding of a treatment plan, a financial arrangement, or possible risks or side effects of treatment, the patient's response is the communication. We all hope that the content of our words is the communication, but it is only the *potential* communication.

The listener, in this example the patient, filters the spoken words, interpreting them through a veil of attitude and interpretation and previous experience and prejudice. Then the listener forms a perception of what was said. Another difficulty with this process is only about 5 percent of the communication is on the conscious level, the other 95 percent is subconscious. So the basic process of spoken communication is:

Spoken word ⇒ Interpretation and Subconscious Processing ⇒ Perception

Another way of looking at all communication is the "S.I.R Principle." This is a rewrite of Skinner's behavioral response theory to include the intellect of the human:

Stimulus ⇒ *INTERPRETATION* ⇒ Response

All communication will follow these pathways, whether oral, written or electronic media. In fact, all information resources suffer the same fate.

Have you read a teen magazine lately? Probably not, unless you have teens in your household. Magazines directed at teens are designed for an intended, specific impact. The messages are "in your face" in ways that make many baby boomers and most seasoned citizens uncomfortable. But the design of the pages are actually an accurate representation of how information enters our brains. The colors and pictures may seem immature to more sophisticated readers, but a teenager can mentally digest one of these magazines in a few minutes with excellent comprehension.

Information is processed through our senses and from there into the brain. Visual learning accounts for about 80 percent of the information we process. Auditory learning is only about 10 percent. But we insist upon most of our communication being oral/auditory. Touch, taste and smell make up the other 10 percent.

In the dental office, patients are exposed to touch in an highly intimate location, numerous clinical odors that are mostly perceived as unpleasant, and powerful tastes that are always unpleasant. These perceptions color our ability to communicate, because the patient's senses are being bombarded in ways normally reserved for more pleasant experiences such as kissing, smelling baking bread, tasting a nice beverage or bite of food. It's a wonder that in the face of all this perceptual noise any of our oral communication gets through.

My friend Marsha Freeman has a saying she likes to repeat: "I know you believe what you understand what you think I said. But I'm not sure you realize that what you heard is not what I meant!" This really describes the confusion that often is the result of our attempts at patient communication.

How can we be certain that our oral communication it is clear? Here are several keys to clarity of spoken communication:

Keys to Clarity:
- Active listening
- Visual aids
- Supporting written materials and correspondence
- Use of electronic instructional media such as Casey™
- Monitoring of results

Let's take each of these in turn, and briefly describe a well designed and effective patient communication program. Later, we'll apply these same concepts to all other office communications. Remember, the purpose of all dental practice communication is to create *positive patient outcomes.* So beginning with the patient communication program makes sense, since all the other communication in and surrounding the office follows.

Listening

Communication is about *listening*, not about *telling*. Effective clinicians get 80 percent of their information from listening to their patients, not from the clinical exam. The data from the clinical exam and objective data simply supports the information already received by the dentist in his or her preclinical interview. Also, presentation of treatment plans and even financial arrangement plans are about listening. If the patients have had the time and opportunity to express themselves and be understood, they are primed and ready to understand what you have to offer in your communication. Active listening is a process that allows you to maximize your communication effectiveness. It is a simple process that occurs in four steps:

1. Listen to the patient, participate in the conversation by making eye contact, nodding and generally indicating your interest.
2. Ask open-ended questions that require other than a "yes" or "no" answer.
3. Verify what you think you heard by repeating back a paraphrased version to the patient and asking for confirmation of accuracy.
4. Clarify the content of what you heard.

You might find it easier if you know how you like to ask for verification, and do it a similar way each time. "It's important to me to be sure I completely understand what you are saying, so I'm going to briefly tell you what I heard." The patient will acknowledge the accuracy or lack thereof, and you can then clarify and confirm with another try at verification. Some other phrases you might choose to use as lead-ins for your verification inquiry are:

> So you feel...
> It seems that you are saying...
> You think, (believe, see, etc.)
> What I hear you saying is...

Using a variety of expressions and statements helps to keep both you and the patient interested and involved in the conversation and avoids a mechanical application of this technique. Dentists are technically oriented and prone to mechanical application of verbal skills. Avoid the temptation to say things only one way. You are trying to enhance your effectiveness with your patients *one at a time*. It is so important to be genuine and truly involved in building a relationship with your patient, and use new communication tools to enhance that process. The relationship you are forming with a new patient is the foundation of success in all future communication and understanding between you and your patient.

When the roles reverse, and you are the speaker or presenter, you can take control of the situation and help your listener become an "active listener." You do not have to teach them a technique or tell them what you are doing. You simply do this by following the same steps, but the roles are switched.

1. Help the patient stay involved by making eye contact and keeping the information brief and nontechnical. Use "layman's terms" as substitutes for all dental terminology. Most patients hear dental terminology as jargon and are offended by it; at least subconsciously they may feel inferior.

2. Frequently ask the patient if he is "still with you," or "clear about what you are saying", just to keep him involved. (He or she will usually say "yes" and it helps keep the person interested.)
3. Use visual aids.
4. When you have finished a complete thought or small segment of your presentation, ask the patient for verification. "It is important to me to be sure that you completely understand what we've covered, so could you please interpret for me what your understanding is of what I said?" Don't make the mistake of simply asking, "Do you have any questions?" after a long explanation.
5. Clarify the errors in communication, then move on to the next point or topic. "That's close, but what *I meant to say was...* " Take responsibility for the missed communication by not implying that the patient heard you incorrectly.

When you incorporate this communication tool in your case presentation for example, two things happen almost immediately. Your presentations are much simpler and clearer, and your patients understand better and accept your advice more readily. The first time you try it you may be surprised at how poorly the patient understands your communication. After verification and clarification, you will be better understood. Then you can make adjustments in your next case presentation to have it shorter, clearer and more effective.

One of the goals of all initial communication and most ongoing communication is to learn about the patient, not just his or her complaint. In order to be understood, you must first learn enough to understand the patient. Information derived from pre-clinical interviews and conversations with the patient during the exam will usually provide enough information to determine the patient's dominant social style. According to Robert Bolton and Dorothy Grover Bolton, authors of ***Social Style/Management Style,*** there are four basic social styles that we will encounter in our practices. Patients and staff will fall into one of the four *styles:* the *Amiable,* the *Analytical,* the *Driver* and the *Expressive.* Each of these types will respond best to communication that is directed to his or her personal social style. In other words, by learning enough about our patients to determine their preferred or dominant "social style," we can better serve them by more effective communication. Here is a brief description of each style:

Amiable: *Relationship oriented, cooperative*

Characteristics—These individuals are motivated by social and interpersonal interaction. They are usually socially outgoing and place a high priority on acceptance, cooperative behavior and friendship.

Guidelines for communication—Do offer personal assurances, expressions of concern and genuine interest in them; have patience in communication; create a feeling that they are valued as people. Avoid seeming rushed, abrupt, rapid, or cutting them off, or pressuring them to accept treatment. Having a domineering attitude or demeanor, forcing communication or patronizing them will be ineffective.

Analytical: *Thinking oriented, cool headed*

Characteristics—Appear cool and independent, even cautious about opening up or extending friendship. They are deliberate, interested in facts and details and like tangible, solid presentations of facts and analysis.

Guidelines for communication—Show them the time and "study" you have made or are willing to make for their case. Be on schedule and respect their time, but allow time for a clear, solid, tangible and analytic presentation of facts. Avoid being disorganized or unprepared, being too casual or informal, especially with information and logic. Do not use opinions or other testimonials to try to influence an analytical.

Driver: *Action and results oriented, risk takers*

Characteristics—Results oriented people, often referred to as "type A" personalities. They tend to be very businesslike and forceful, and very direct in their communications. Time oriented.

Guidelines for communication—Be clear and specific. Be brief and get to the point. Give an organized, logical and efficient delivery of services or information, and ask for a decision. Avoid trying to establish a "personal" relationship, personal or folksy conversation, and wasting time. Don't make decisions for them.

Expressive: *Intuition oriented, creative*

Characteristics—Imaginative and creative, they are often spontaneous and even flamboyant. They are the least disciplined of the four styles in the use of time. Outgoing, playful, and full of energy, they are quick to make decisions and dislike routine.

Guidelines for communication—You need to have time for socializing and listening to their personal stories and opinions. Plan on giving a written report formalizing the details, since it is often hard to achieve a focused presentation or conversation. Avoid being seen as abrupt, cold or autocratic. Do not appear prejudicial or judgmental or overly task oriented.

Once you have identified the social style of the patient, record it in the patient's chart and share it among the staff. If the staff and the doctor are all consistent in their efforts to communicate with the patient, then this process will not appear manipulative or mechanical. Again, the purpose of all dental practice communication is to create *positive patient outcomes.* If your goal is personal success and financial prosperity, the patients will feel your insincerity, and these methods will undoubtedly fail.

Visual Aids

Communication delivered visually is better understood than spoken communication received by auditory sensation. Visual aids can range from the simple to the complex. As a general rule, a patient should be presented just enough information in all forms to satisfy his or her need to understand the information being presented. An analytical needs more logical information presented very carefully and logically, and an amiable needs less analysis and more demonstration that the doctor and staff care about him or her as a person. Visual information can come from many sources. I suggest all of the following be available, but do not necessarily use them for every patient:

- Actual pre-treatment Kodachrome photos of the patient
- A photo album of actual patients' before and after photos (used with permission)
- An intraoral camera for on-the-spot visual aids. May also be used to provide for video stream or printed still images for a later consultation
- Casey® or other interactive video instructional program
- Brochures and booklets describing procedures

With each of these available, the doctor and staff can determine the social style of an individual patient, then plan and prepare the necessary visual aids to have on hand during the case presentation. When questions or concerns arise during the course of treatment, the same approach can be made, selecting just the right visual for the patient's style.

The Importance of Persuasion

It is your goal to educate your patients and bring them to a high level of understanding of their personal dental conditions. Another important goal is to inform them of the marvelous treatment available to provide remedies for these problems. Finally, for any of this effort to matter at all to the patient or the doctor, the patient must accept the treatment plan, make a financial arrangement to pay for it, and proceed to treatment.

Most management companies today give seminars on "selling" dentistry to patients. Certainly case acceptance is the ultimate goal of a clinical case presentation. But it is not the only goal. Educating your patients, demonstrating their needs clearly and simply, and informing them of the scope of therapeutic practice you have available in your hands to fulfill the needs of their case are the primary goals of a clinical consultation. Yet, without the ability to confidently persuade patients to accept treatment, all is lost. The clinical information may as well not have been given.

Most sales courses teach the same theories and practical applications. The elements of influence that are typically presented are *"logic"* and *"emotion."* These are taught by seminar leaders and management companies all over the country, and many dentists have taken such classes and heard how to apply the theory. People, whether consumers, clients or patients, are said to base their buying decisions on emotion, and will support their decision with whatever available logic is provided to justify the decision. So the theory is to find the emotional "hot buttons" that cause the patient to be moved, and use them to close the "sale." Hot buttons include both positive motivators such as health, beauty, function or "saving money," and negative motivators such as avoidance of pain, great financial expense, inconvenience. The emotional element is presented first, in the form of *benefits* tailored to that particular patient's motivators. If you address the emotion in a form of a benefit to which the patient readily relates, then you may have his or her attention. The logic is presented second, in the form of a *procedure,* which describes the rational and technical procedure offered as a solution. So the formula becomes "*Benefit plus Procedure*." You may have heard the terms.

There is danger hidden in this formula. Because this technique is often mindlessly and mechanically applied, it may come across to the patient as a very transparent effort to get him to "buy." It therefore reduces your (hopefully) carefully planned and very personal clinical service to a commodity, and the patient becomes a consumer. Transforming a potential *patient* into a consumer of dental commodities is precisely what you want to avoid! Consumers are ferocious animals, prowling the earth for the best buy, undiscerning of quality, out to save a buck.

Patients confronted with a poorly delivered sales presentation that is not focused on their needs and appears in any way insincere are naturally suspicious and untrusting. The doctor is reduced to the level of any other salesperson, and the patient assumes the role of a skeptical *potential* buyer. In a professional practice that delivers highly specialized and personalized health care services, much more is expected. You are a doctor, not a merchant of fillings, and discerning patients have high expectations of your clinical competence and professional demeanor. This does not include the casual application of mechanical selling techniques in case presentations.

The five keys of a successful clinical case presentation are sincerity, preparation, simplicity, clarity and persuasion.

Sincerity means you are truthful, genuine, and possess the knowledge and skills to perform the procedures you offer to a high standard of practice. You are open and willing to give of yourself, to communicate who you are, and reveal your true personality and commitment to the patient. It comes across loud and clear to anyone with whom you speak, and requires no special effort for case presentations. But if you don't believe in yourself and your own abilities, how can you be sincere with your patients? Be sure you have the skills available for the procedures you offer.

Preparation means having the patient records available, along with all the graphic information discussed elsewhere in this chapter. I like to review the case well in advance of the consultation appointment, usually the day before after the conclusion of my clinical day. It is essential to call and discuss with the selected specialists any specialty issues that are not clear. Review the anticipated treatment plan, and the patient's progress to date. In essence, have the personal and clinical observations and information about this patient clearly in mind. Use models, X-rays and images as support.

Simplicity is important because patients do not have our scientific and technical training. The concepts, terminology, and technical knowledge we take for granted as dentists are beyond even the most intelligent patients. One of my friends is a professor at our local university. He is a bright, intelligent and articulate scientist and an excellent communicator as a teacher and dean. He taught me a wonderful lesson. He became a patient and as we began our clinical discussions, I assumed he wanted a lot more of the technical and scientific basis for all that I do. I gave him lengthy explanations and detailed rationales for all of my considerations and determinations for his case. After several visits, we were tasting wine together in his home, and he commented that he could not understand how I was able to get such high case acceptance, since I spent so much time trying to explain things to my patients that they really can't understand anyway. I said, "But you mean my *other* patients." His reply was very revealing: "No, I mean *me.* I don't understand half of what you say to me in the office because the dental vocabulary you use has so little in common with mine!" He went on to ask that I communicate the procedures and rationale in detail, but to eliminate the dental jargon. Our professional relationship was extremely successful thereafter, and he went on to complete a very complex comprehensive treatment which included some endodontics, two years of orthodontics, four quadrants of periodontal surgery and a full mouth reconstruction. I tried to never use a dental jargon around him again. It was good to be reminded, since I had weaned myself off "dentalspeak" years before for all but a few select patients, primarily analyticals who seemed to pick up the vocabulary. Though now I doubt that they truly understood it all. I thereafter quit "using" at all and give up my addiction to dentalspeak..

Review and even rehearse privately what you want to communicate to the patient. Make it simple, and eliminate any technical words that have plain English substitutes. Say "decay," not "caries"; "jaw joint," not "TMJ"; "destructive bite" instead of "malocclusion." Don't talk down to people. Just help them understand by avoiding ambiguity and confusion.

Clarity goes along with simplicity. Say what you mean in plain English or plainly in your common language with your patient. Mean what you say, and do it with clear verbal precision. Then frequently ask for confirmation from the patients. When they can accurately relate back to you the essence of your message, you know you have connected. If you use dental jargon, they will not be able to relate back the information.

Case acceptance is highest when the patient completely understands the important features of his or her own case. So use all of the tools at hand to communicate using the various senses. Pay attention to the Five Keys to Consultation discussed above. Show tooth models and images to the patient. Use before and after case studies. Let the patient hold and feel his own models and models of completed work similar to his treatment plan. I like to use enlarged models to demonstrate tooth contours. The patient can feel the various planes, angles, dips and doodles of a 10X central incisor, and it helps him appreciate the precision and quality of your work. Describe how he will feel, how comfortable their function could be, how pleasant things will taste and smell, and how happy he will be to display a really beautiful smile. Mention the compliments he will receive from his spouse and close friends. Sight, sound, touch, taste and smell may all enter your discussions at appropriate moments.

Persuasion is the final key to successful case presentations. Here theories of sales methodology that include logic and emotion do come into play. As you can see, much of the material presented and discussed above applies to both informing and persuading the patient. The theory of "emotion plus logic," which is the basis for most sales courses originated with Aristotle, and has been passed along in various forms for centuries. But somehow in our consumer culture a major part of the Aristotelian essence has been lost. Aristotle referred to not two, but three "proofs," or elements of proof. These are *ethical, emotional and logical* proofs. The reason many sales pitches are so offensive is the salesperson fails to establish the *ethical proof* before proceeding with the emotional and logical proofs. This is also the reason most post-management seminar dental consultations seem like transparently insincere and manipulative sales pitches. If we are to achieve 90 to 100 percent success in case presentation, careful attention must first be paid to the ethical proof.

Ethical proof is difficult to achieve upon first encounter. Ethics refers to character, and character of the doctor must somehow be demonstrated to the patient to establish a relationship of trust. It is not something most human beings grant another upon a first impression. This is one of several reasons why I have never advocated immediate case presentations after short exams. It fails in two proofs. One, the ethical proof is not established by a first impression, even a positive first impression; and two, the logical proof is less credible when based on a cursory examination that is not supported by other sensory materials. Personally, I could never get all the data straight in my own mind so quickly that I could give a complete and erudite case presentation chairside on exam day.

Carefully developing patient-centered relationships gives the doctor the opportunity to demonstrate sincerity, competence, caring and trustworthiness without making premature, overt and arrogant claims to those positive traits. The ethical proof of persuasion is the *rightness, correctness or truth* of the product of the doctor's mind—the diagnosis and treatment plan. You may be believed because you make claims of believability or take some type of an oath, or you may be believed because you are worthy of being trusted by that particular patient. The ethical proof can only be made one patient at a time, and the sum of your ethical proofs becomes inseparable from your reputation in the community.

Supporting Written Materials and Correspondence

Written material is better understood by most adults than the spoken word. In fact, the oral communication is better understood if *preceded* by the written. This is not always possible in the dental office setting, but mailing some information to new patients has some benefit. Also the use of interactive video educational materials in the reception area can prime patients to be receptive to information about their own oral health circumstances. But most supporting written materials will come after the initial exam, since it is impossible to determine in advance what information the patient might need. Here are some supporting written materials for patients:

- Office brochures
- Treatment plans
- Treatment sequencing and appointment information
- Brochures and procedure summaries
- Letters to inform and reassure the patient

As a general policy, the following materials may be incorporated into the information flow for new patients:

1. A new patient welcome package that includes
    - An office brochure welcoming the patient
    - Health history and insurance information
    - A map and written appointment confirmation
2. When the patient is examined, appropriate clinical brochures should be available, especially for the analytical to take home after the exam.
3. At the treatment planning consultation appointment, the doctor should be prepared with:
    - Written treatment plan
    - Phases or suggested phases on separate sheets
    - Appointment sequencing
    - Written consent form if needed
    - A written financial arrangement agreement
4. Following the consultation, a letter may be sent to the patient to list the findings, and confirm the agreed treatment plan. This letter can also be used to reassure the patient of the value and wisdom of his or her decision.

5. During treatment, especially treatment lasting over a period of several months to years, the doctor should send a letter periodically updating the progress, reassuring the patient, and expressing gratitude for his or her continued commitment to health.

Use of Electronic Instructional Media

This is a relatively new form of communication in dental offices. As more patients have become users of electronic media in their homes and workplaces, this tool has taken on new importance in dental offices. The perfect office video communication program has yet to be developed. Here are the criteria that I would like to see in an office instructional video:

- Inexpensive
- Easily installed and updated
- Uses readily available equipment
- Can be accessed from multiple sites in the office without moving a cart
- Written in simple, non-clinical language
- Clear, attractive visual images that use actual case images only for before and after comparisons
- Colorful and clear, non-threatening animated graphics for procedure descriptions
- Fast access between frames and subjects
- Interactive for patient control
- Able to incorporate doctor's material to customize the presentation

Short of the above criteria, there are several interactive instructional video systems on the market. It can be a valuable tool for visual enhancement of patient education.

Monitoring Results—The Patient Survey

Treatment plan acceptance and patient retention in the practice are two simple, easy indicators of effective patient communications. Excellent treatment plan acceptance is acceptance in the range of 90 percent or above. Patient retention is demonstrated by a monthly increase of total patients, a positive net of new patients minus departing patients.

In addition, profitable, effective practices must monitor their patients by survey annually or at least bi-annually. There are several surveys that are published and available for use. A useful sample questionnaire is found in ***Standard Marketing Procedures for Dentists*** by Gordon Burgett ©1997, Dental Communication Unlimited. This questionnaire can be applied as an in-house questionnaire or a mailed survey. The limitation of all self-administered questionnaires is that you have no way to validate the information, nor can you compare your practice with others. Even so, it can be a valuable tool to obtain basic data from your patients that will help to correct areas where you may be less effective than you hoped and intended.

An excellent survey program which I recommend is the ***Patient Satisfaction Survey Program*** from the L.D. Pankey Institute for Advanced Dental Education. This is a quality service audit designed and administered as a collaborative effort of the L.D. Pankey Institute and the Gallup Organization. It validates the accuracy of your practice survey information and compares your results with the top practices in the study.

Patients leave dental practices for many reasons. Every time it is offered, the *Patient Satisfaction Survey* provides fascinating and surprising results:

- The majority of patients leave practices due to a lack of trust, caring concern and friendliness.
- The practices that scored the highest in the bi-annual survey were rated higher by patients in the areas of cleanliness, ease of communication and pro-active patient communication.
- Employees are included in the study, and rated the best practices much higher in the areas of personal development, encouragement of quality work and respect for employees.
- The top practices are the ones that are the most profitable. They enjoy the highest rate of referrals and experience the most substantial loyalty among the patients and the staff.
- The survey measures the areas of *Impact, Trustworthiness, Relationship, Respectability, Accessibility and "Gestalt."*

To my knowledge, the L.D. Pankey *Patient Satisfaction Survey* is by far the best and most complete dental patient survey ever offered. It is available from Dr. Richard Green, Director of Business Systems Development, The L.D. Pankey Institute, 240 Crandon Blvd., Key Biscayne, FL 33149, telephone (305) 361-5433. As a communication development tool, this survey is unsurpassed.

For a comprehensive internal and external marketing program, consult the text, ***Standard Marketing Procedures for Dentists*** cited above.

THE COMMUNICATION PROCESS — Beyond Patient Communication

Communication with Specialist or Referring Doctors

Once excellent patient communications are in place, the positive effects can be undermined if communication standards do not extend beyond the doors of your own practice. Patient communications are about establishing and maintaining relationships. The same can be said for specialist/referrer relationships. My confidence level goes way up each succeeding year I continue to use the services of the same specialists. We have a record of success and achievement that is founded upon years of mutual respect and *communication.*

Referring patients to a specialist should not be an act of simply casting them out to the street to seek out care as best they can. Every dentist should have a selection of prescreened and preferred specialists to give to the patient. The specialist should have very clear, written knowledge of the practice philosophy of the referring doctor. In addition, very complete patient information needs to be transmitted by the referring dentists and received by the specialist before the arrival of the patient.

A referral should have several features to enhance the patient experience:

- A request for a well-defined service or set of services
- A briefing on the patient's medical history, especially highlighting those areas of special attention such as the need for antibiotic chemoprophylaxis
- A dental history and treatment plan in the referring office

- A statement of the referring doctor's expectations of the treatment, a description of the expected end-point of referral services

This is *not* to say that the referring doctor can *demand a particular* outcome he or she may desire. Many specialty procedures are less predictable and can have a range of acceptable results. This communication should provide a summary of the treatment plan, a reasoning why the specialist's services are needed and the desired outcome and benefit to the patient.

Expediting Specialist/Referrer Communications

Establishing a definite referral network has enormous advantages for both the patients and the doctors. Predictable outcomes, ease of communication, trust and respect are achieved only by well established referral relationships. The first step is to decide whom among the available specialists a referring doctor would like best to have as a partner in clinical care. Then arrange a meeting between the specialist and the referring doctor. The meeting has several purposes:

- Open lines of personal communication with each other.
- "Interview" the other doctor to see if your philosophies are similar.
- Share the written *Practice Philosophy,* and ask for input from the other doctor to see if the doctor is aligned with your practice philosophy.
- Begin to establish the foundations of mutual understanding that will lead to the trust and respect partners need to achieve their best results.

Following the initial meeting, doctors who are interested in forming a working relationship need to meet at least one more time. The purpose of this meeting is to discuss the practice philosophy presented during the first meeting, and to see if each practitioner is willing to undertake a collaborative effort to refine the individual practice philosophy into a mutual statement of philosophy that will guide their relationship. This is really a "position paper," a statement of philosophy that defines the relationship and the expectations of each party. It is not a formal contract that defines obligations. It is a statement that establishes guidelines for success for patient care and for the long-term relationship between the practices. This important communication within the professional team does not replace spoken contact. It covers certain foundation issues such as:

- A statement of practice philosophy from each doctor
- A description of the key benchmarks of hospitality issues will be handled in the referred-to practice. Key modalities such as how individualized attention to the patients' personality or social style will be provided, how the patients' schedules will be accommodated, how behaviorally appropriate patient management techniques will be applied. Even such detail as how the phone will be answered and how the patients will be greeted should be considered in this paper.
- Expectations of treatment plan information and how it will be conveyed
- Follow-up expectations, both for the patient (will they be called the evening after the day of surgery) and for the referring doctor
- A discussion of mutual beliefs on current treatment modalities and technology

- An agreement about the particular philosophy of patient relationship as the basis for patient care
- The paper should be as specific as possible, pronouncing agreement or consensus on all major beliefs of the practices, including such things as occlusion, centric relation, splint therapy and equilibration. The role of the specific specialist in providing certain service should be defined: Does the periodontist provide the "night guard," or does the generalist provide "occlusal splint therapy? Does the orthodontist "adjust the interferences" after appliance removal, or does the generalist remount the case and do trial model equilibration and final clinical equilibration? Is the object of periodontal surgery in the anterior region a perfect attachment, or will surgical technique have an eye to finished esthetics?
- Identification of key issues will indicate those areas of harmony and agreement. It will also reveal areas requiring modification or enlightenment of deficiencies if the patient is to receive coordinated services resulting in optimum patient care.

This collaborative effort, and the position paper produced, will enhance the achievement of specific patient outcomes to obtain optimum health for the patients.

Establishing Referral Pathways

Referred patients are always a bit apprehensive. They have placed a great deal of faith in the decision to refer. These patients hope that the specialist they meet will be an open, friendly, technically competent doctor with an equally friendly and accommodating staff who are well trained and efficient. The referral method that they encounter at the referrer's office, and the statements made about the specialist practice go a long way to establish the relationship of trust and understanding we have been describing. An excellent referral has several important features. It must be an endorsement of trust, faith, confidence and recognition of the benefits of a long term successful relationship between the practices. The referring doctor must confer confidence in the specialist and relate personal knowledge of many successful outcomes in similar patient circumstances. Yet the referral must not imply a promise of success. It should not interfere with the specialist's professional prerogative, nor should it obligate either doctor to a particular outcome. Let the specialist do his or her own analysis and appropriate informed consent.

Developing close referral relationships requires time and effort. The result is often a smaller group of more exclusive referral associates. This is ultimately a big benefit, since the effort required to build the understanding and appreciation between the doctors yields continuous and ever improving rewards in optimum patient outcomes with the added benefit of ease of communication increasing office efficiency.

The patient is not *required* to follow your referral recommendations. If they choose to go outside of your team, then see if you can communicate with their chosen specialist. Share your treatment plan and all information of previous treatment and intended future treatment. Try to get the specialist to read your *Practice Philosophy* and a position paper from a member of your referral group in the same specialty. Who knows? You may end up with an excellent new addition to your ensemble!

There is risk to the patient seeking a specialist outside of your resource group. These should be carefully explained to the patient without being judgmental of either the patient or the proposed specialist; basic ethical considerations demand nothing less. Remember he or she may be a rising star who will ultimately be on your team! I prefer to engage the patient in a conversation that lists and reviews the *benefits* of seeing my preferred specialists, and leave it at that. In 20 years of clinical practice, I have had several occasions where the patient wanted to see a personal friend, a fellow church or club member or a relative. You risk undermining your trust and credibility if you push too hard on these issues. Informed patients usually make excellent choices. Always support whatever their choice—it is the best one for them at the time.

THE FIVE C's OF COMMUNICATION

Communication in any form has five requirements to be effective. It must be:

1. Clear
2. Concise
3. Contemporary
4. Complete
5. Confirmed

Precision in dentistry is essential to success. Communication can be no less precise when the subject is the dental care. Plan your communication and base it on the treatment plan and previous treatment. Be ***clear*** in your own mind what you want to accomplish, and clearly communicate this to your colleague.

We're all very busy, and ultimately all this effort invested in communication procedures should pay off in time and efficiency. Be ***concise*** in your communication. Brief, well thought-out communications are preferred and appreciated.

Timing is everything. Your communication must be ***contemporary.*** By that I mean get it delivered as soon as you have clearly and concisely defined the need. A message delivered to the orthodontist the morning of the new patient exam is too late to be of value.

Though brief, make an effort to be ***complete.*** Try to formulate a complete, comprehensive communication and deliver it. You can then clarify with brief follow-up discussions. But if the basic message is strung out over several different communications in as many different forms, you can bet the message received is not the one you intended to send.

Confirm your communications. Call and ask your colleague if he or she received your letter or memo. Are there any questions? Ask them to repeat to you the essence of your communication to confirm you are both "on the same page."

ACCEPTABLE PATHS FOR COMMUNICATION

Written communication is usually better than oral when multiple issues are to be covered or a single issue is complex. It is generally more clear, concise and complete. It is easy to confirm. The major problem is making it contemporary. In a busy practice it is a problem to find sufficient time in a day to complete all the written communications necessary. Fortunately, there are solutions to this problem:

- Develop form letters for routine communications
- Use prepared templates on your word processor for addresses and formats
- Use macros or memorized segments to reduce time per letter
- Save previous letters for reference

All letters should be from one doctor to the other. Other than dictating content, it is unwise to delegate clinical communications.

Telephone communications are excellent and sufficient for many short and single-issue communications. Letters and e-mail are useful for communicating treatment plans, case histories, problems and concerns regarding a referral. They are also best for certain patient communications such as a follow-up to a treatment conference and for an annual update on findings or progress. But the telephone is really the instrument of choice for many important patient and specialist communication. It is the marketing lifeline of the practice. In most practices all appointments not made in person are made and confirmed by telephone. Initial introductions and appointments to specialists can be by phone. Post-treatment calls to the patient the evening of treatment are the only way to have a timely communication.

But the telephone has some traps that can create all sorts of havoc with risk management. Many offices have the routine wherein the dental receptionist calls the specialist office to make an appointment and request a service. One auxiliary or unlicensed clerical worker is talking to another. The medical-legal requirements for a referral are not met. If the referral is then followed by a written prescription, signed by the referring dentist, then the loop is closed and everyone is fine. Or are they? Often, the prescription is also prepared by the receptionist or other assistant, and simply signed by the dentist, if at all. Specialists must then decide if they need to follow-up with a call or if the referral is sufficiently complete. Training and professional experience never make a receptionist on either end of the phone into a qualified decision-maker for patient care.

Communication Tools

The referral slip is a basic and effective communication tool when properly used. It should be completed and signed by the doctor. If delegated, or dictated or completed by an auxiliary from the treatment plan, it *must be reviewed* and signed by the doctor prior to delivery to the patient or by mail or FAX to the specialist. You may prefer to use slips developed in your practice to communicate *your* desired services and outcomes. This should be determined while producing the position paper.

Letters and memos, whether mailed, FAXed or e-mailed are by far the best form of treatment plan communication. Clear, concise and complete, they provide the least opportunity for error. Make them contemporary and then confirm, and you have the potential for perfect communication.

Clinical Planning Meetings

Some of the most fun and rewarding moments of professional life can occur during planning conferences among your team of specialists. These meetings should be formal enough to result in a written summary report of each case in which the specialist will participate. More about this in the next chapter.

Following this chapter are *Standard Operating Procedures* for:

- Patient surveys
- Developing a position paper

PATIENT SURVEY

[patsurve.frm]

Desired Outcome: To conduct periodic polls of our patients to determine the satisfaction level of the patient population to enable us to make correction in our methods and procedures.

Measurement: Information provided by polls is applied to our standard operating procedures to create improvement in the subsequent poll.

Steps for conducting a patient survey:

1. Determine areas of inquiry and create appropriate questions, or

2. Review the previous survey and adjust or repeat the questions as necessary.

3. Randomly choose 100 patients to whom to mail the survey.

4. Select 100 patients to whom to mail the survey.

5. Leave 100 survey forms in the reception area.

6. Mail the 200 surveys with postage paid return envelopes. Use a mail service so non-returned surveys do not cost postage.

7. Allow two weeks for survey returns.

8. Tabulate the results.

9. Review the results of the survey at a staff meeting.

Patient Survey / 2

Note: The ***Patient Satisfaction Survey*** conducted semi-annually by the L.D. Pankey Institute Business Systems Development Department and the Gallop Organization is the best way to conduct such a survey. In the years between, you could conduct an abbreviated survey to address those areas which your previous survey identified as areas of undeveloped strengths that need attention.

POSITION PAPER

[positpap.frm]

Desired Outcome: Create a position paper stating the essential philosophy of this practice as it relates to specific specialty providers.

Measurement: Efficient referral communications and successful patient care outcomes in our interface with selected specialists.

Name of specialist ______________________________
Date ________________
Specialty ______________________________________

Frequency of referrals ____________________________

Steps for production of a mutual position paper:

1. Establish a meeting with the specialist and the referring doctor.
2. Interview the other doctor to open lines of communication and establish areas of philosophical agreement.
3. Share your written Practice Philosophy with the specialist. Describe it orally, and provide a copy for him or her to read.
4. Follow this meeting with a telephone conference to discuss your philosophy and the specialist's response to it.
5. Arrange for a second personal meeting.

Position Paper / 2

6. At this meeting, propose and deliver a statement of practice philosophy which incorporates your views on specialty care for mutual patients. This document needs to have certain elements:
   - A statement of philosophy from each doctor.
   - A description of hospitality standards for the offices.
   - Communication standards, including forms which will be exchanged, and expectations for telephone consultations and follow-up.
   - A general statement on current standards for treatment and technology applications.
   - Philosophy of patient relationship.
   - Clinical philosophy.
7. The position paper is left with the specialist for no more than two weeks for review and editing. Telephone contacts are made to discuss points of view and mutual desires.
8. A final meeting is held to review the finished document.
9. Review is held annually or more frequently as needed.

Chapter 7

PATIENT-CENTERED COMMUNICATION

Nothing is standard in the treatment planning business. Many dentists believe that it is in the best interest of the patient to withhold most of the information the dentist has gleaned from his exams. These doctors pulse information and recommendations to the patient over time—here a filling, there a root canal, here a crown.

Over time the patient has a considerable amount of dentistry completed, but at a standard far below what can be achieved with the technical sophistication available today. The dentist looks in the mouth and tries to find something overtly broken or decayed. Ignoring the more subtle signs of deterioration such as wear facets, cervical abfraction defects, periodontal lesions unexplained by oral hygiene, incisal chipping and wear and a myriad of joint signs, symptoms and sounds, the dentist goes merrily on his or her way supervising the slow erosion of the dental health of the patient. Just give the patient a "check-up," institute a "Soft Tissue Management Program" and find something restorative to do. These nearly random "what's worst today" decisions are within the so-called "standard of care" created by the insurance industry and supported by peer review. Unfortunately, these decisions lead to treatment that cannot possibly be completed in centric relation. Each restoration is created to replace the role of the partially malfunctioning natural tooth or previous restoration it replaces. Unhappily, the slow iatrogenic changes that occur as a result of the small errors incorporated into the occlusion of random restorations completed over many years can lead to significant pathology of the temporomandibular joint and the muscles of the head and neck. It is likely that, if the patient lives long enough, there will be a need for total replacement of all the previous restorations with attention to centric relation occlusion, occlusal-muscle dysfunction, TMJ considerations and periodontal considerations.

Many business management consultants support this model. Their goal is to maximize "production" as a measure of practice success. Individual patient care is given all the nice "buzzword" attention, mainly to create a marketing image. Hygiene departments are supposed to become "efficient." Hygiene income is targeted at some 30 to 35 percent of the total office gross income. Soon, the heart of the business of dentistry is centered on the doctor's prosperity, not the patient's well-being. "Patient reactivation," "Accelerated Hygiene" (sometimes under the guise of "Soft Tissue Management") and "Cosmetic Dentistry" are often substituted for a missed understanding of comprehensive patient care.

It has been proven in studies of actual dental practices conducted at the L.D. Pankey Institute that an emphasis on quantity, reactivation, acceleration and other "volume" concepts does not create the most profitable practice. The pace of the practice and lack of close patient relationships can lead to rapid professional burn-out. In fact, the most profitable practices have hygiene departments that produce in the neighborhood of 20 percent of the total office income. This allows the doctor time to spend providing quality services to fewer patients.

When asked, many doctors confess they are afraid to perform complete exams and present comprehensive treatment plans because they fear the patient's rejection. They may have had patients decline their initial efforts to practice in this way, and have now adjusted to a briefer, less comprehensive approach. Or they lack confidence in their own diagnostic and restorative skills and have achieved a comfort level for their practice. Others erroneously believe that if they have an extensive, detailed treatment plan, they are under some moral, ethical or legal obligation to complete it.

What is in the best interest of the patient? The next section will help sort out some of the complexity of treatment planning. It will suggest ways to organize the findings and engage the assistance of your colleagues to enable you to implement treatment plans that keep the patient's optimal health at the heart of the process.

The Treatment Plan

Treatment plans are comprehensive, written documents that communicate the total plan of treatment as it is understood when the plan is written.

Notice, I didn't say the plan must be completed on the first visit. Nor did I say that the *initial* plan itemizes all the dentistry the patient will ever receive or outline a plan for lifetime optimal health. That may be possible in some cases, but in others, the initial plan, *when written,* may be a very simple document. It takes a bit more time and effort with examination and diagnosis to arrive at a comprehensive treatment plan ready for presentation to the patient. Let's look at an example:

Mary White is a 42-year-old mother of three who recently presented for a new patient exam. She heard about new bleaching techniques and wants her "front teeth to look better." A summary of her exam findings includes recent TMJ clicking and masseter muscle pain. She has excellent oral hygiene and has regular visits for dental prophies all her life.

You note that she has noticeable upper incisor shortening, numerous wear facets, and other signs of occlusal breakdown. She has some isolated sulcus depths of 5-6mm. You record numerous broken-down amalgam fillings, and three over-contoured PFM crowns which are violating the biologic width on first molars.

Mary's treatment plan will eventually call for replacement of the PFM crowns and the amalgams. It will address her cosmetic complaints and bring her to optimal periodontal health, and it will definitively treat her TMJ pathology, not just wait for it to become bad enough to refer to someone else. But the initial plan we will present today is designed to deal with the problems that need to be solved first. So it may detail the need for an occlusal appliance to diagnose and stabilize her occlusal-muscle problems and help diagnose her TMJ dysfunction, recommendations for imaging of the joint, a referral to our periodontist for evaluation and treatment planning and a consultation.

It is important at this stage to begin a relationship with Mary that will grow and mature over time. Our immediate goal is to learn her dominant social style, find out how well she understands her dental health, help her visualize and understand her oral condition, and to define the outcomes that she desires. Is she most concerned about the esthetics of the short anteriors? Does she understand why the gums are red and bleeding around the crowns, even though she takes special care to clean those areas? Does she want to have optimal periodontal health and keep her natural teeth all her life? Is she concerned about the joint problems?

By identifying the problems, not as a disinterested or aloof academic doctor, but as an interested care-giver, we begin to engage Mary in a process of co-diagnosis. She becomes involved in the treatment planning, and the need for manipulative or mechanical sales techniques dissolves in the warmth of a genuine relationship of trust. It may take a great deal of time over many visits. Or it may come quickly, but the relationship is the basis for treatment acceptance.

Our initial plan in this case is:

1. Complete TMJ Imaging series
2. Mounted Study Models
3. Consultation
4. Trial Equilibration on Models
5. Occlusal Splint Therapy
6. Referral to Dr. Larson for periodontal evaluation.
7. Specialist conference with Dr. Larson

The next steps that I would anticipate at this time would be written in a "Phase 2" plan:

1. Remove PFM 3, 14, 30; replace with properly contoured custom acrylic provisionals
2. Re-evaluate biologic width 3, 14, 30

By involving her in a process of co-diagnosis, Mary will have an excellent idea of the problems we encountered in her exam. If we address her needs using the communication guides to her *Amiable* social style, we will be able to gain acceptance of the treatment plan. As we learn about Mary and get more examination information from the progress of the splint, we will be able to refine and develop the next phases of treatment.

It may go something like this:

Phase 3:

Upon recommendation from Dr. Larson, we will:

1. Remove PFM 3, 14, 30; replace with properly contoured custom acrylic provisionals
2. Dr. Larson will complete the following procedures in her office:
    a. Root planing procedures

b. Periodontal crown lengthening procedures and grafts in UL, UR, and LL quads

Dr. Larson will remove the provisionals to help with access and replace with our specified provisional cement after surgery.

Phase 4:

Occlusal therapy is complete, and periodontal procedures are successful.

1. Equilibration
2. Restore anteriors with ceramic crowns to establish, color, contour and anterior guidance.

Phase 5 and beyond:

Restore posterior teeth in segments according to logical sequence derived from analysis of individual tooth conditions.

Patient finances and insurance issues are the common barriers dentists feel prevent them from practicing excellent clinical dentistry. By building relationships with our patients, these problems are more readily solved. Patients who do not trust you or value your opinion and who have not been part of the exam and decision process will refuse treatment over their insurance limits. Our goal is to create a sincere relationship of trust, then work to find ways for the patient to afford the services.

What do we accomplish by hesitating to move swiftly and make six anterior crowns to answer Mary's chief complaint? After all, they were covered by insurance, and we know *"cosmetic dentistry"* is what patients want, right? By hesitating we were able to diagnose the occlusal problems that caused the wear in the first place. By correcting that first, we will be able to provide ceramic veneers or crowns that (1) won't break, chip and crack like her natural enamel did; (2) provide proper anterior guidance to protect the TMJ and the posterior dentition, and (3) look fantastic—because when the criteria of both form and function are achieved it becomes possible for the dentistry to be exquisitely natural in appearance.

So, take into consideration patient finances and availability for appointments. The patients will understand this to be part of your commitment to them.

For most patients, the initial treatment plan is a step to building a comprehensive treatment plan. We learn about our patients as the relationship grows, and our goal is to *ultimately* provide a comprehensive solution to the patient's oral health needs. Each phase of treatment has the following treatment plan features:

- Written
- Sequential
- Number of appointments and approximate length
- Diagnosis for insurance narratives
- Specialist services identified and listed
- Fees and insurance estimates
- Date diagnosed
- Date completed

The Specialist Conference

Early in the treatment planning process, specialist conferences provide the missing link to many clinical solutions. Integrated into the treatment planning process, specialist conferences can prevent missed diagnosis and wasted effort from misdirected attempts to treat complex problems. A specialist conference can be a meeting with the one specialist whom you need to assist you with a particular case, possibly a periodontist or orthodontist. For more complex cases, a group conference is very effective.

Your team of specialists can be your most valuable clinical and educational resource. Specialist conferences should be initiated by the general dentist, though they are usually initiated by the specialist after seeing the patient. For best results, a clinical conference should occur early in the treatment planning, and as early as possible in the patient relationship.

Here is the way we have seen the best clinical success in specialist participation with cases: Gather together whenever is necessary to review cases in a study club format. Bring your newest cases—those being processed through the clinical exam sequence. You can hold the meetings in the conference room of one of your offices, but the location may be anyplace where four or five doctors can gather, show slides and pass around models.

Call your orthodontist, periodontist, oral surgeon and endodontist if necessary. Review cases that are to involve *more than one* of the specialists, but it is not a requirement that each case involve all of them. Few cases need that much specialist attention. There is tremendous benefit in having them all attend. The summed experience of all the doctors in the room is enormous, and valuable contributions are made by individuals even when they will have no particular role in a given case.

In a short and efficient evening you can review and treatment plan four to six cases. The referring general dentist should be the scribe, taking notes to later process into a comprehensive, phased treatment plan. If the general dentist's clinical records are comprehensive, the patient need not have been examined by each specialist prior to the meeting. If office location and logistics allow, you may even want to schedule certain patients for short sessions with the entire group. The specialists will have a very clear idea of the patient and the goals of treatment after the meeting. They can then see the patient and deliver a completed treatment plan and narrative to the general dentist before the general dentist arranges a consultation with the patient to present the treatment plan.

Some conferences do not bring major breakthrough discoveries. They are valuable nonetheless. All conferences result in a treatment plan that is more comprehensive and tailored to the individual needs of the patient.

The Treatment Referral

Referrals may be for evaluation and consultation, or they may be for specific procedures, such as a particular endodontic procedure or a crown lengthening surgery on a particular tooth. If treatment planning and sequencing is performed as recommended above, the specialists are aware of the case and communication is already established. The specialist will be expecting the patient and ready to provide the services previously planned.

However, sometimes things aren't so smooth and predictable, and the patient has a new or emerging need that wasn't previously addressed. The communication then becomes a *Treatment Referral* which should be as accurate and complete as possible.

The *Treatment Referral* includes the following information:

1. Patient name
2. Referring doctor
3. Brief history of complaint with relevant treatment history
4. Available images, photos, even study models can be helpful, if available
5. Specific procedure requested
6. Intended treatment to follow in referring office

The referral should be completed by the referring doctor, or if dictated, reviewed and signed by the referring doctor.

Objectives and Outcomes

The standard of care throughout the nation now generally requires that a treatment plan be made, in written form, that communicates to the patient and future providers a corresponding treatment for each problem identified in the examination and diagnosis. This plan needs to be clear, and though not necessarily sequential, needs to set some sort of priorities for ordering treatment.

The Issue of Consent

Like a written treatment plan, informed consent is a standard of care throughout the nation. It may be given orally, but the prudent doctor presents treatment both orally and in written documentation and has the patient sign a "consent to treat" form. Though it has been said that this consent does not necessarily provide the doctor with legal proof of such consent, it at least establishes the fact that the patient had the opportunity to read and review the plan. Consent may then be proven by other means.

Most malpractice lawsuits are not won or lost on the issue of consent. It has a much greater bearing on actions by regulatory agencies directed against the doctor's license to practice. The fact that the *routine* in a practice is to obtain a signed consent from the patient goes a long way to demonstrate the standard of care in practice should the issue ever emerge regarding insurance company reviews, state board actions or civil litigation.

A note on creating your own forms and letters

This is a brief discussion of the standard operating procedures theory developed by Marsha Freeman.[1] Standard operating procedures are useful here to provide a protocol for making your communications formal and predictable. Referral communications need to be exceptionally clear to provide optimal care and avoid liability. The chapters that follow will provide information for communications between general practitioners and their selected specialists, including laboratory communications. Each chapter will discuss some of the special challenges encountered with each relationship, and how to best organize your communication to meet those challenges.

Creating a referral standard operating procedure or "SOP" is a simple process. There are three features of a typical SOP:

1. A **Desired Outcome**—a brief description of the goal of the procedure, task or document.
2. A **Measurement**—how you will recognize success.
3. A set of **clearly defined tasks**—usually a series of steps or a description of the task.

In the case of referral procedures, each type of referral requires its own SOP. We will see how these operate in the ensuing chapters that deal with each specialty specifically.

The Desired Outcome of most referral communications will have three basic goals. The first is the patient-centered goal of having the *reason* for the referral clearly communicated. The specialist may be called in for a variety of reasons, and it really should not be his or her problem to figure out

[1]From ***Standard Operating Procedures for All Dentists*** by Marsha Freeman, 3rd ed., 1998. See last page for details.

why. The second goal is to provide a communication link for the record. The third is to avoid liability for error or negligence. The desired outcome should be clear and concise.

Measurable results are described in another simple and concise statement. The results are specific to the task. Look for specific results for each type of communication. In any case the results should have an outcome that is observable, measurable or quantifiable.

The tasks are defined in a series of steps that allow the desired outcome to occur in a way that can be measured. This should include any forms or communication documents or guidelines used in your office for referrals.

A useful checklist for completion of a communication SOP is:

1. Is the task clearly defined?
2. Is the SOP easy to read?
3. Is its objective clear?
4. Do you understand the procedure described?
5. Are the responsibilities precisely stated?
6. Is the process clear and logical?
7. Are there any gaps, assumptions, leaps of faith?
8. Does it solve the problem? Or does it create other problems?
9. Does it provide for enforcement and discipline? Establish policy?
10. Does it reference any standards, laws or regulations?
11. Is it numbered and clearly identified?
12. Is it in a standard format?

Use details of *who, what, why, where, when, how* the referral or other communication will be completed. There should be sufficient information that the entire task or process can be readily understood by a new employee or substitute who will use the SOP as a guide.

Following this chapter are standard operating procedures for:

- Referral protocols
- Planning a team treatment study conference

REFERRAL PROTOCOL

[refprot.frm]

Desired Outcome: To ensure that all referrals made from this practice are made to selected specialists, in an efficient, complete and timely manner.

Measurement: Efficient referral communications and successful patient care outcomes in our interface with selected specialists.

Steps for referring a patient for specialty examination or treatment:

1. Doctor (only) diagnoses the patient condition and determines the need for referral.

2. Doctor identifies the specialist to whom the referral is to be made.

3. Auxiliary staff do not determine the need for referral, nor to whom the referral is made.

4. The referral is formalized on the appropriate **Specialty Referral** form, filled out and signed by the doctor.

5. Doctor will indicate any special conditions circumstances on the referral slip.

6. The form is an NCR triplicate. FAX the top copy to the specialist, then mail the actual top copy to the specialist, or give it to the patient to take to the specialist if the visit is today.

Referral Protocol / 2

7. Place the middle copy in the patient's chart.

8. Place the third copy on the doctor's telephone "IN Box."

9. Doctor will telephone the specialist as soon as possible whenever deemed necessary.

10. Doctor will describe any exceptional circumstances in an immediate telephone consultation when necessary.

11. The specialist may call to confirm the diagnosis and treatment plan, to report on the procedure, or to question the doctor about special circumstances. Such calls are reason to interrupt the doctor.

TEAM TREATMENT STUDY CONFERENCE SOP

[studycon.frm]

Desired Outcome: To ensure that comprehensive, state of the art treatment is provided in a multidisciplinary approach, using teams of selected specialists.

Measurement: Efficient clinical communications and successful patient care outcomes in our interface with selected specialists, in a team approach for comprehensive multidisciplinary clinical treatment and follow-up.

Steps for forming specialist teams:

1. After enrolling specialists in the cadre of selected specialists, choose a case involving more than one other specialist, such as a periodontal prosthesis case involving periodontic and orthodontic specialists.
2. Prepare all records necessary in your office to perform diagnosis and treatment planning.
    - Kodachrome slides or video
    - Articulated study models
    - Clinical records
    - Mock up (wax-up) of case goals
3. Have the auxiliary staff arrange a meeting at your office or one of the specialists' offices.
4. The meeting time and date is confirmed with the selected specialists.
5. Before the meeting, the slide projector and video monitor are made ready, and the records are displayed on the conference room table.
6. Coffee and soft drinks are made ready and available 15 minutes prior to the meeting.

Team Treatment SOP / 2

7. The patient coordinator attends the meeting to record minutes of the conversation.
8. Doctor will dictate a letter outlining the comprehensive treatment plan determined as a result of the conference.
9. Each specialist will submit a written treatment plan for their service area to each other and to your office for permanent record.
10. Our office thereafter provides tracking and clinical coordination of procedures for the patient.

Chapter 8

CREATING POSITIVE PUBLIC PERCEPTIONS

Public acceptance of dentistry has never been better. Today, dental health is seen as an important element of a successful lifestyle by 70 to 80 percent of the American public. Yet many negative perceptions remain in the way the consumer of the twenty-first century views the profession of dentistry, and his or her experience of being a dental patient. These negative perceptions cause responses from mild anxiety or nervousness to complete avoidance of the dental experience. Overcoming these negative perceptions is a key to a successful dental practice.

Messages that consumers receive from advertising and the information media are potentially inconsistent with the actual consumer experience in dental practices. Certain marketing messages are particularly misleading, especially when issues of "quality" are advertised to the public. For example, many of the large HMO clinics recognize that the dental consumer has no accurate way to evaluate the standard of care or quality of service an individual may receive. They also recognize and take advantage of the fact that "quality" has no definition in dentistry and can be freely used as a marketing term or buzzword. "Quality" in these environments has come to mean or imply dentally insignificant features of the practice such as adequate parking, reduced waiting time on telephone hold, convenient hours, on-time appointments, easy appointment availability and little reception room waiting time. "Quality" is assured, they proudly tell their clients, by an internal "peer review" or "quality assurance" process that may involve nothing more than an annual spot check of charts for completeness. But the public has no meaningful way to interpret any of this information. They respond to marketing images in much the same way no matter what the subject. If the message "resonates," "hits a hot button" or somehow emotionally connects with a person, they may act or respond to the information. If not, the message isn't really even heard.

Major changes in marketing and patient perception threaten the small practitioner. The high volume clinics are backed by significant capital resources. Some new modes of practice involve schemes to have national franchises of dental "brands" through management organizations with huge financial resources backing them. This first appeared in orthodontic practice, where the franchise practices market orthodontic services directly to the public, eliminating the step of a general dentist referral. These practices do not develop any referral relationships with area dentists, preferring to market directly to the public and through their existing patients. The consumer enticement is price. They will do any case for an advertised monthly fee.

"Patients won't stand for that!" you say? "They'll see beyond the hype when they experience the poor quality of the service," is another common protest from dentists. But wait: what does the patient find in these organizations? Does she enter the practice only to be disappointed that the radio feature does not describe the reality? The answer is "no." The potential patient finds exactly those features that resonate "quality" to the average American consumer. The office is in a convenient location, near work or home and easily accessible by automobile. There is lots of parking, in a well kept, landscaped lot. The entry way and door is shiny and clean.

There is a pleasant, well-groomed receptionist with a ready smile to welcome her to the office. The reception room is airy, light and very clean with beautiful colors and textures of fabric and finishes. There is soft music that the patient finds familiar, but cannot identify. The new patient forms are simple and clear. The patient is escorted through her entire experience in the office by a pleasant, friendly and professionally groomed assistant. The doctors are very efficient, seem not to be rushed, and listen and answer questions. They defer most logistical questions to the support staff. The examination and record taking processes are smooth and seem efficient. Consultations, typically with an assistant, are quick and direct. Treatment plans are simple and clear. There is ample time for questions. Financial arrangements are as advertised—one fee for any service in the orthodontic example—but clear and firm in any case. Throughout the entire experience, the patient hears her name being used. On the first visit, each patient is offered a tour of the office. At each visit the patient is treated like a guest and is offered refreshments such as coffee and juice.

There are two different and *independent* quality measures in any business. Customers, clients, or patients make decisions based more upon *perception quality,* which is the evidence of quality available for the observation or perception of the customer. Perception quality includes such things as cleanliness, order, hospitality, friendliness, ease of purchase, service (as in table service or personal attention from an agent of thc businccss), pcrsonal attcntion and general attention to visible, tangible details. Banks were once masters of perception quality, since their service was really intangible. Clean branches, marble floors, high ceilings, attentive tellers. Today, with mergers and high speed electronic banking, the perception quality has moved toward marketing style and consumer convenience. Replacing banks as the standard for perception quality are the highest quality hotels and restaurants. In a dental office it is the patient journey, or subjective experience of the office environment, hospitality, ease of treatment, ease of financial arrangements, convenience of location and hours of service and personal attention of the staff and doctor.

The other quality is performance or conformance quality. Conformance quality refers to the actual performance or character of the product or service itself. It is a measure of whether the product of service meets or exceeds either an expected quality standard, or one declared by the provider of the product or service. In the case of a fine resort hotel, it is the fact that the stay you enjoy is entirely relaxing and comfortable, with no hassles or inconvenience. Your room is clean and ready, the view perfect, and you enjoy a quiet and luxurious stay. In the case of a dental practice, it is the actual quality of the treatment, the achievement of comfort, function, harmony and longevity. It is quality materials, well trained professional staff and qualified doctors.

What is a patient to believe? Are there any clues to a lay person that the services provided by the clinic described above are definitely not customized to his or her personal needs? Does the patient have any way to evaluate the clinical ability of the doctors with whom he has the most superficial relationship?

It appears that the patients do respond to these environments in a very positive fashion. They believe the *evidence* of quality from the surroundings—*perception quality*—carries over to the quality of care—*conformance quality*. Once they have entered and been dazzled by the *hospitality* of this new office in town, little can be said or done to get them to leave. Especially if your office is the typical private, solo practice...

Solo practitioners have operated for years under the assumption that the patients will continue to seek their services because they somehow understand that the "quality" is better in the fee for service private practice. They rely on the ability of the patient to *detect* the superiority of the services they receive, or to *understand* it is better because of the sincerity and integrity of the doctor. The doctors assume their *conformance quality* will somehow find its way into the patients *perceptions.* Even practices that try to teach the patients about the quality differences risk sounding arrogant or self-aggrandizing. So "quality" is something dentists must simply just *project* or *transmit.* We had better hope all the patients are tuned in to receive these messages.

Solo fee-for-service practices have a hard time competing with the acquisition of technology that volume clinics are able to afford. This is a great time in history to be a practicing dentist. New technology is exploding, providing clinical benefits for patients at an unprecedented rate. Intraoral video, lasers, air particle microabrasion, interactive video education, operating microscopes, fiberoptic illumination, precision instrumentation, computer graphics and communication tools are all adding value for the patients and complexity to the practice. Modern consumers expect to see new technology, and believe it to be superior to the old. When they find it in a clinic, they believe it confirms their choice. And the volume clinics are filled with the obvious signs of new technology.

Practice survival into the twenty-first century in the fee-for-service arena requires each practice to communicate benefits of its practice to its patients and to the community in direct, visible, objective and tangible ways that demonstrate features modern consumers perceive as "quality." In other words, when we communicate "quality" we need to do it better than anyone else, and in ways the public can recognize.

The first step is to be sure each of the hospitality features described above is met in your office. From the first phone call to the follow-up after treatment, are you exceeding the hospitality offered by the "clinic" you disdain? Matching their perception quality only levels the competitive playing field.

The next step is to exceed each patient's expectations of communication, clinical service, administrative efficiency and personal follow-up. It is not enough today to simply greet and seat, provide treatment and dismiss. The patients who remain with you and refer others are not the ones who were just satisfied, but *completely* satisfied. Any office can learn to meet the highest expectation of hospitality. Restaurants and hotels do it routinely with less educated and less talented staffs. Learning to provide equivalent levels of *clinical and administrative* proficiency that patients feel and communicate to others is a more difficult task.

Complete satisfaction will not be judged by the perfect shade match of your porcelain veneers or the undetectable margins of your onlays. This is unfortunate, because *clinical ability* is reflected in *conformance quality,* and really is what objectively separates the finest practitioners from the volume operators. Patients benefit from superior services by accuracy, comfort, function and longevity of the service. But patients cannot discern this very well, at least not for many years. Many doctors think it is enough to spend some time with the patient up at the end of a visit and simply tell him what a great job he or she just did. This method has obvious social pitfalls. Some patients will be receptive and respond in a positive way. Others will find the doctor arrogant or self-aggrandizing, or perhaps a brash and uncouth braggart. Still others will wonder why this is needed at all, expecting each procedure *should* go perfectly.

Patients will judge the clinical quality the same way they judge the practice hospitality—by the performances of the key players in the drama and by the surroundings. To be seen as clinically proficient, the clinical team must practice together in a way that is viewed as smooth, efficient, calm and controlled. The drama of the dental appointment can be made negative or even frightening by barked commands, frustrated responses and negative interactions between the doctor and the clinical staff. Making the doctor or the patient wait, being left alone in the operatory, or not having instruments and supplies on hand, are all readily observed mistakes that patients do notice. Alternatively, a dental patient can experience the dental appointment as a calm, well planned, completely organized, predictable and even pleasant experience for operating team. It can be made to be humorous and even fun!

Patient perceptions of administrative accuracy and proficiency carry equal weight in patient satisfaction. If the general hospitality was perfect, and the clinical procedure went without a hitch, but the administrative assistant is edgy and demanding, and financial arrangements are not clear, the credibility of the doctor and the practice is severely undermined. After a clinical procedure, a lengthy and confusing financial discussion will destroy any memory of the operating team's prowess—and any previous confidence of quality. The patient will leave angry or frustrated, with a predominant recollection of the unpleasant exit procedure. He may even tell a dozen or so friends and colleagues. The irony of the independence of perception quality and conformance quality has struck again. The patient can leave the office with the finest crown ever made and yet be disappointed with the result!

Quality is communicated through caring. Two minute follow-up calls *by the dentist* to check up on the patient are worth more in patient trust and assurance than *any* in-office communication. Thcsc calls can be made in the afternoon to morning patients, and immediately after dinner in the evening to the afternoon patients. Post-op calls are made to assure the patient that the doctor cares enough to follow through with his or her commitment to the patient; it assures the doctor too, that the entire visit, in fact, went well. Patients always react positively to clinical follow-up, and if you take the time, you will receive valuable information feedback on where to improve your practice.

Dentists think of dental services as tangible pieces of "work"—a surgery, a veneer, a crown or a resin filling. They believe if they provide that service to perfection each time they perform it that "quality" has occurred, and *somehow* the patient will understand that fact.

On the other hand, patients see dental services as a *journey* through your office. They share an experience with your team, exposing an intimate part of their body to relative strangers, trusting that you care enough to do a good job. Patients see the weeds in the landscaping and the cobwebs in the corner. They notice the only time you failed to wash your hands *in front of them* and the assistant with an obvious cold. They sense any tension in the interpersonal interactions of the staff and especially the encounters with the doctor. Dental visits are tiring, and the last thing most patients want is to have a demeaning financial discussion when they really would like to leave.

A better journey for a patient is to arrive at a pleasant office, be addressed by the staff and the doctor in a friendly and courteous fashion, have the clinical procedures completed efficiently and without discomfort and have a brief and pleasant financial exchange and reappointment upon exit. Then, to the delight and often amazement of the patient, a follow-up call from the doctor "just to see how well you're doing," seals the conviction that this is a quality practice.

Success is an enormous challenge. The office must guide a number of patients through this journey each day. Success requires total commitment and focus on the details from the doctor and the staff. But it does not require a superhuman effort, nor does it require perfection. Often dental offices are likened to athletic teams, and teamwork is emphasized using athletic metaphors. We have "morning huddles"; the doctor is the "quarterback"; we ask hygienists to be "team players." How does this view of the patient journey, with its incumbent requirement of near perfection and attention to detail fit in with a team model? How can any staff ever be so perfect? It seems that we fail if we make a single error!

Think of your staff as a volleyball team. At any moment it may seem quite chaotic. But look around. Players are getting into position, anticipating the needs of others and the unpredictable flight of the ball. And someone always comes through to *keep the ball in the air.* Never let the ball touch the floor, at least not on your side of the net. That is the goal of volleyball—and dental practice. Yet sometimes the ball does hit the floor. The goal is to have that happen as seldom as possible. Successful teams are the ones that make the NCAA tournament, or win it. Very few balls hit the floor on their side of the net over the course of the season. Those teams who make so many errors that the ball often hits the floor on their side are the losing teams.

From the time each patient first calls the office to the follow-up phone call, and then each time the cycle repeats itself, *never let the ball hit the floor.* If it does, *immediately reorganize* to get the service back. *Get the service back!* When you have failed to keep the ball in the air, it is not the end of the world, and it happens to the very best teams in every match. The successful ones immediately recover, *get the service back*, and go on without looking back.

Get the service back. You know when the ball hits the floor. It is no use to stop everything, do a post mortem on the error, chew someone out, or otherwise dwell on mistakes. Do what it takes to correct the immediate error. Be sure to recognize it and apologize if necessary, but do move on. You have many more opportunities to demonstrate hospitality, clinical proficiency, administrative proficiency, and follow through yet to come. There may be more opportunities for superior performance with this very patient. And there are more patients scheduled who are just beginning their journey.

Take advantage of those developing opportunities, and in the long run, you will have a winning team.

The way to beat the competition and survive and prosper in the future is simple. Create a nexus of conformance quality and perception quality for each patient in your practice 100 percent of the time. The "pigeons" and "shorebirds" can't do this because they will never achieve the conformance quality of the best clinical practitioners. The Eagles and perhaps the Songbirds must merely learn to pay attention to perception quality and deliver top quality services.

Chapter 9

SYSTEMS AND THEIR APPLICATION

Systems and their implementation

Though this is not a book primarily about systems, the subject needs introduction and discussion to complete some of the important processes of practice design. After communications failures, systems failures are probably the second most important cause of practice failures, so the subject is extremely important. Yet there is a lot on systems in the literature and the consulting marketplace, so I do not want to repeat much of that here. Therefore, I will present a condensed version of *Systems Theory* and *Systems Implementation* in order to provide a cohesive and integrated approach to your thinking about *Designing Your Perfect Dental Practice.*

Consultants and Advisors

At the outset, let me say that nobody has a perfect set of systems that you can buy and drop into your office. Numerous failures and even bankruptcies have been the result of misguided efforts to make the systems' foot fit the dentist's shoe. Remember the cliché: "When all you have is a hammer, everything looks like a nail?" Management companies abound, each with a "patented" or "copyrighted" set of systems. Many are based upon a single premise, such as "patient reactivation," "recall" or "expanded hygiene," "soft tissue management," "esthetic dentistry," "laser dentistry," "microdentistry" and the list goes on... Others are based upon a new and sexy popular trend in the business management press such as "downsizing," "management by objectives," "re-engineering," or some popular psychological theory or social science theory. Most if not all of these "secrets" and "discoveries" have some value. The problem is how does a practicing dentist evaluate, choose, hire, and implement such a program? And why limit it to a fad? Why try to become a nail because somebody brings in a hammer? (You might rather be a brick.) There is huge risk, especially when the management companies will only tell you their success stories. Plus, the costs have risen exponentially.

I hired my first management company to provide systems training and implementation in my practice in 1984. The cost was about $4,000 for a year of monthly meetings, plus my staff's free attendance to any classes the company gave. We attended four seminars and a small workshop during the year, and they came to my office for about a half day each month. It was a fair value, and we learned quite a bit. Three years later we hired them for quarterly visits for a higher cost, about $6000; no seminars were included. Today such a service ranges from about $25,000 to $40,000, and few actually come to your office. A bit more of an increase than inflation would account for? You bet.

Can you simply do it yourself? Probably not. In my experience you can save yourself five to ten years of grief and accelerate your practice development in equal measure by getting professional help with your management dilemmas. My personal bias is to hire a consultant who can provide some personal evaluation and assessment, and will address your specific dilemmas over a period of 12 to 18 months. I also feel office site visits, meetings, and workshops are more effective than large seminars. When a Fortune 500 company hires a consultant, the consultant usually provides services at the corporate site. They seldom require the corporate managers to come to them.

There are four types of consultants.

♦ The first is an *expert* consultant. This is a tax attorney, your accountant, a real estate broker or financial planner. You seek their services for a specific need they can address. You *could* do it yourself, but it would take an enormous amount of time and resources, you do not have their training and expertise, and ultimately, it would cost you more money.

♦ The second kind of consultant is a *training or technology* consultant. This is the person you hire to bring new technology or techniques to your company. In the management arena, it may be the consultant who helps you and your staff to implement a new computer system, management system or new technology or equipment. They may stay a day or several days over a period of time. They may facilitate a staff meeting or work with an individual.

♦ The third type is the *process* consultant. This person can deal with the entire range of specialized expertise in their field. It is one who can assist a client in improving the status quo in a number of ways, applying specialized knowledge, expertise, skills, content, behavior and contacts to create the outcome. They facilitate staff communications, help design and implement business systems and organizations and help with strategic planning.

These folks are the best value, because their impact is dramatic. But it does not happen in seminars, it happens at your office.

♦ The fourth type is a *compliance* or *dependency* consultant. This is a consultant who in essence takes the place of some functions you, a manager or another employee should be doing. They usually provide some data management or monitoring and teach their own system without customization; however, they add little or no expertise, technology, content, skills, knowledge, or behaviors to improve the practice. They fill a niche in the operation of the office that makes the client reluctant to end the relationship. They sometimes seem inexpensive compared to other consultants. But remember it is a relationship which won't end until you fire them. Until then you'll pay a lot each month for little value.

Costs for these categories vary within and between categories. In general, the first two are the least expensive, primarily because they are the most limited. The third is probably the most beneficial. But this is a hard area to evaluate, and there are a lot of posers who are willing to take your money. The fourth I don't recommend in most circumstances. Try to get training to replace any long-term monitoring or compliance "consultants" with in-office procedures. All your long-term advisors should fall into the first three categories. Pay them when you need them, and get periodic "tune-ups." In between, it feels good when things are running well.

Systems Theory

Systems theory is really a simple concept. The purpose of management systems is to provide a structure for the numerous tasks and duties, which are categorized into logical groupings. The groupings, their names and content are not terribly important. I'll give some examples below. Consulting companies all try to put their own "spin" on the systems they teach. But the result is largely the same, whether the company has four systems or 104 systems. (It is a true story—one company I know claims to have 104 "systems" they teach their offices. I'd hate to be the person keeping track of *those* monitors each month.)

Within each "system" there will be a group of tasks that need to be performed, and some measurable way to monitor the outcome or completion of each of those tasks. The measurable results are gathered daily, weekly or monthly in a simple format to report the outcomes. These monitors are also called different names such as "monitors," "indicators" or "variances." It is helpful if the monthly indicators can be contained on a single page that tells the summary version of the practice performance that month. To be complete, systems are not just a list of the tasks. Systems include the guidelines for the outcome of the task, the mechanics of how to complete the task, the necessary activities and behaviors to be successful and the monitors or indicators for checking the outcome.

Too few systems makes each one cumbersome and illogical. Too many and the effort to run the systems overwhelms the benefits. So the middle ground is best. I prefer systems theory that creates about ten to 12 systems, with subgroupings within the systems. Here is an example of how you might want to structure your systems:

Dental Practice Systems

1. Financial Systems
    - A. Financial Arrangements
    - B. Collections

C. Accounts Receivable
D. Insurance
E. Payment Methods

2. Scheduling Systems
A. Communications
B. Organization of the Book
C. Productivity
D. Mechanics

3. Recall and Hygiene Systems
A. Continuing Care
B. Hygiene Department
C. Scheduling
D. Periodontal Maintenance
E. Management
F. Compensation

4. New Patient Systems
A. Communication
B. Moments of Truth
C. Exam
D. Patient Records
E. Treatment Planning
F. Consultation
G. Financial Arrangements
H. Scheduling
I. Follow-up

5. Budget and Inventory Systems
A. Cost Categories
B. Budgeting Process
C. Ordering
D. Controls

6. Marketing Systems
    A. External Marketing
    B. Internal Marketing
    C. Communications
    D. Budget
    E. Planning

7. OSHA and Compliance Systems
    A. OSHA
    B. CDC
    C. Local Compliance Requirements
    D. Infection Control
    E. Radiation Safety
    F. Employment Guidelines
    G. Training

8. Patient Education Systems
    A. Staff Training
    B. Hardware and Software

9. Facilities Management Systems
    A. Daily Operations
    B. Weekly and Monthly Operations
    C. Budget
    D. Maintenance
    E. Refurbishment
    F. Furnishings and Fixtures

10. Personnel Systems
    A. Finding and Hiring
    B. Training
    C. Staff Meetings
    D. Conflict Resolution
    E. Team Building
    F. Morale

G. Performance Reviews
H. Benefits
I. Termination

11. Monitors and Business Indicators

Each of these systems must be adapted to the *Practice Philosophy* instituted by the owner and the staff. Difficulties emerge when an office attempts to apply an alien set of systems without regard to the current culture and history of the office. So get help, but don't buy somebody's turn-key systems package for a lot of money. If you have great systems in place that are working, chances are your culture is already defined. So get it all in writing in order to keep it consistent over time and when training new staff.

The next step of business organization is the extension of the *Practice Mission Statement* into various forms of practice philosophy. Practice philosophy is the translation of the mission into the myriad activities that occur during the day to day operation of the practice. It controls and directs the daily activities from the moment the door is open and the lights are turned on, through the many interpersonal encounters with patients and staff, to the locking up at night.

Hiring a Consultant

Business systems are the mechanical tools that define day to day operations of a business. Business systems are essential for the success of any enterprise. They spring from the vision of the practice, and therefore the practice mission. Systems are the operational guidelines for the management of the practice, and provide the recipe for daily, weekly, monthly and annual procedures.

They are also an area of considerable debate and confusion among dentists. Business systems must emerge from the vision and mission of the practice or they will be irrelevant to the operation of a particular practice. This is one reason why the millions of dollars spent by dentists on "practice management consultants" is often wasted. If your practice mission happens to fit the systems of the particular company you hire to "consult" with you, then success may be achieved. But if you do not fit their mold, the result will be a poor fit and lots of wasted time and money. Some of the management companies even want to give you a new vision of religious truth, as well as their particular version of management reality. Others are equally dogmatic about applying their particular "principles" of business management.

This is not to understate the importance of business systems, but to emphasize the importance of tailoring your systems to the requirements of your particular practice mission. Not all, in fact very few, management consultants are capable of doing this. So be careful in your selection! Having said that, let me also state that most practices cannot design and implement a complete set of customized financial, business and clinical systems without the assistance of a competent business consultant.

The steps I use are by no means unique, but may serve as a model to use while interviewing consultant candidates. My preference is to begin by selecting a consultant who has license to use Marsha Freeman's Standard Operating Procedures technology from Dental Communication Unlimited. DCU certifies professionals to apply the SOP format to your practice and produce a set of completely customized systems to fit your vision, mission and philosophy.

A true consultant is much more than a "management systems teacher." Many programs are simply educational in nature, some better than others. Consultation involves much more. A true consultant must be a very dynamic person who is a very perceptive analyst, an experienced planner, with an ability to collaborate and communicate. He or she must have a thorough understanding of the business principles that must be applied to produce and help you implement your operating systems.

The consultation must begin with some sort of systems or operations inventory. I use two forms of discovery to assist in my initial analysis. The first is the *Practice Needs Assessment* that identifies, assesses and rates all the existing systems or lack of systems in the practice. This is used when the practice is not in a current crisis, which is rare. When a practice is in some sort of operational crisis, the proper entry level assessment is called a *Critical Issues Analysis.* This analysis seeks to identify the critical issue or issues that are causing the current breakdown of operations in the practice. Solutions are created by collaborative effort, and implemented as fast as possible. After the crisis has somewhat quieted, the *Practice Needs Assessment* can be carefully completed.

The next steps are to help the doctor or doctors articulate a vision for the future of the practice and distill that to a mission. Then the mission is carefully applied to each system in the practice and a written set of procedures is completed to produce a predictable, stable *Business Format.* This format uses *written documentation* of all the policies and procedures used in the operation of the practice. In a way, it is a set of guidebooks that could be applied to recreate *this exact practice* anywhere, any time. It is used to integrate the various functions of the practice and to train and orient staff. The documents included in a completed Business Format include:

- Statements of Mission and Philosophy
- Standard Operating Procedures Manual
- Personnel Manual
- Regulatory Compliance Manual
- Financial Management Manual, including at least three years of history

Each manual is a working document that can be reviewed and modified as often as needed. My preference is for a multiple three ring binder format, with the above titles. Each page can be saved as a word processing document in your own computer system for easy editing and updating. This business format is itself a system that integrates all the elements necessary to make the practice run smoothly. It transforms a chaotic, complex environment into one that runs like a machine, or like a self-healing organism. The establishment of systems that are designed and implemented to achieve your singular goals, creates integrity of the seemingly unrelated concepts of patient care and financial management to achieve incomparable results.

The Entrepreneurial Dentist

Sounds like a good piece of work, doesn't it? It is. But it is also the path to predictable success for the dentist who has both clinical skills and an entrepreneurial spirit, the one who wants to succeed by helping people. Most dentists are capable of at least average clinical results. The key element of successful dentists is that they all find ways to create a business to support their clinical efforts. The difference between a mere clinician and an entrepreneurial dentist is one of perspective.

The mere clinician has no passion for the enterprise itself, and expects the practice to produce a personal result—income for the doctor. The entrepreneurial dentist sees things differently. He or she views the business as creating a system for providing external results for the patients, with the result being profits. The irony is that the clinician works more selfishly for personal results, and the entrepreneur works to create excellent external results for others, and thereby profits. This necessarily requires a broader, more futuristic vision with an intention to create systems to change the present into that future vision. The practice must be viewed in its integrated form, all the parts in systematic relationships to one another. The mere clinician sees the practice in a fragmented, disintegrated way, with each part a potential problem or crisis. It is easy to see that the mere clinician is very vulnerable to the intrusion of managed care, since the mystery of the business systems overwhelms his or her capability to integrate the systems into a business format. This is the clinician who dreams about "just doing dentistry" and will ultimately sell out to a dental management corporation. The entrepreneurial dentists understands that his or her fate is better mastered than forfeited; he or she works to achieve the integrated vision of practice that creates profits by providing for patient needs.

Which will it be? Each of us must choose, but systems are not the burden. Creating customized systems is a lot of work, and is not without frustration. The integrated systems of the entrepreneurial dentist are the path to clinical and economic success. The results are the realization of your dreams.

Chapter 10

SCHEDULE BUSTERS: COMMUNICATION WITH YOUR ORAL AND MAXILLOFACIAL SURGEON

Many general dentists enjoy surgery. Some of them are quite proficient at it. Few are very efficient, and fewer are fully equipped to handle difficult cases or sudden complications, nor are their staffs adequately trained and experienced with complications.

From the patient's perspective, there is no other referral that brings more obvious benefits than a referral to an oral and maxillofacial surgeon (OMS). An OMS offers surgery, conscious sedation, ambulatory outpatient general anesthesia and a variety of inpatient and outpatient hospital procedures. OMS residencies include training in medicine and surgery, most with three or now more typically four years of hospital training. Some OMSs have earned a medical degree and have completed medical internships and are licensed to practice medicine. They have skills in general anesthesia that provide enormous comfort and benefit to the patient that few general dentists can provide. They have advanced training in their surgical specialty that surpasses that of a surgically trained dentist such as a graduate of a General Practice Residency or

Advanced General Dentistry program. Their offices are equipped with more advanced anesthesia, patient monitoring and cardiac life support equipment than most general dental offices. They are efficient and expert in their procedures and have specially trained support staffs.

The busy general practice may have several reasons for requesting consultation and treatment of a case by an oral surgeon:

1. The patient has high anxiety.
2. The patient is medically compromised creating greater risks.
3. The patient requests general anesthesia.
4. The doctor doesn't perform the procedure.
5. The procedure is unpredictable in the general dentist's hands.
6. The scheduling is unpredictable.
7. The procedure has developed since the doctor was trained.
8. The procedure requires special equipment.
9. The patient is in pain, or there is likely an infection; it is an emergency.
10. The oral surgeon did four of these yesterday. The last time the referring doctor did one was a year ago.
11. Standard of care and liability considerations dictate referral.
12. The specialist's office is better prepared to evaluate and treat a patient that is at high risk for transmission of infectious diseases.
13. You demonstrate concern for the comfort and well-being of the patient, and enhance your image with your patient and his family by referring the patient to an expert.

But the two big reasons are numbers 3 and 6 above—*patient requests for general anesthesia,* and *surgery wrecks your schedule.*

Special problems exist when considering surgical treatment requests. Oral surgery offices are different from general dental offices. The oral surgeon gets his referrals mainly from general dentists and occasionally other specialists such as orthodontists. He or she probably does not have a written practice philosophy and must meet the expectations of a large number of referring doctors. The offices typically have a less "patient-friendly" feel, being much more clinic-like or even hospital-like. Some, *but clearly not all,* oral surgical staffs have an inflated opinion of the dental specialty social hierarchy, or the perceived value of the services performed there, and may act somewhat superior. Patients are seen only two or three times—for exam, surgery and post-op—and are not considered important referral sources in the unenlightened practice. Out of practical necessity, many oral surgery offices also see an abundance of social welfare cases. This, plus the need to weave significant numbers of emergency referrals into their carefully scheduled day may lead to full and chaotic waiting rooms. Patient hospitality can be a much lower priority than in your (now) carefully crafted office environment.

Of course, there are exceptional and enlightened oral surgeons who recognize that what they do reflects favorably or unfavorably upon their referring doctors, and have created environments as carefully designed as the best general practice. Make your life easy, and find one who has done the work to create an office atmosphere that most closely mirrors yours. If you cannot, then you have the option of using the tools provided in chapters four, five, and six to formulate a mutual practice philosophy that addresses the issues of coordinating your hospitality, clinical proficiency and administrative proficiency with the other practitioner. There is no easy way to fulfill this mission short of putting in some time individually over the table with your chosen specialists. It is sometimes difficult to inspire change in the unwilling, but the rewards are worth the effort. You will be helping your patients and yourself by influencing the surgeon to create an environment where the patient you refer will not only receive the care you intended, but will experience a level of personal attention, hospitality, clinical expertise, and follow through consistent with *your* mission statement. The surgeon will benefit as well, through increased referrals from other conscientious general dentists, from improved patient outcomes and increased patient satisfaction.

First, let's consider routine referrals for elective surgical procedures. The surgeon needs to know:

1. Personal data about the patient. Name, address, telephone.
2. Significant medical history that may influence treatment. Not a narrative of all positive and negative findings; simply alert him to potential problems—diabetes, liver disease, heart disease, etc.
3. Known indications for chemoprophylaxis
4. Any known allergies
5. The procedures you are requesting. Be specific. It is wise to include a method to have a fail-safe description of teeth to be extracted. Redundancy is indicated here: Chart the teeth, indicate the tooth numbers in writing, and verbally describe them. ("upper right lateral incisor, number 7," and "X" it on the chart)
6. A time table for your treatment plan. Are you waiting on this procedure to proceed with another? Do you need this to be done before a second specialist provides some treatment? Or is your treatment complete, and this surgical treatment can be done

purely electively, i.e, third molar extractions "this coming summer." Do you need to coordinate insurable benefits with the surgeon?

Routine referrals need a standard communication protocol. Having your receptionist call the surgeon's is not sufficient. It does not provide adequate contact between the doctors and exposes each to a heightened risk of liability. Though this may be a standard routine to get the patient scheduled, it does not constitute a proper request for treatment. The referral protocol must include some written or oral contact between the two doctors, preferably both. Here is a sample of the requirements you may want for your referral protocol:

1. Dr. General, the general dentist diagnoses the need for a surgical treatment and documents it in the patient record. She decides to refer the patient to Dr. Surgeon.
2. Assistants do not determine to whom the patient is referred.
3. The referral is formalized on a standard form, completed and signed by the general dentist. (Staff members frequently make errors on these forms. Don't take the chance of being liable for a staff error. Simply fill them out yourself.)
4. The form is an NCR triplicate or is copied for the record.
5. The form includes all the data listed above.
6. The receptionist or patient coordinator assists the patient with making an appointment with the surgeon's office according to mutually developed protocols.
7. The patient retains a copy of the referral.

8. A copy of the referral is mailed or FAXed to Dr. Surgeon.
9. Dr. General may call and briefly describe the referral to Dr. Surgeon during the telephone call period within 24 hours, if necessary or if the case is not routine.

If the referral deviates in some way from the routine:

10. Dr. General will either write or dictate a referral letter to Dr. Surgeon detailing the specific circumstances of the request. Usually documentation includes the patient's detailed medical history and treatment plan for exceptional consultations.
11. In cases of multiple specialties, special cases like cleft lip/palate or challenging reconstruction or implant cases, a meeting between the doctors is indicated.
12. The more complex the case, the greater the need for additional face-to-face meetings for both case planning and progress reports.
13. In all complex or non-routine cases, after exam and prior to treatment, Dr. Surgeon will telephone Dr. General to confirm the diagnosis and report on the scheduling for the procedure.

There is an important caveat from the perspective of both the surgeon and the patient. General dentists often feel that they need to "make a case" with the patient for referral. Many patients do initially express some anxiety about having to go somewhere new and unfamiliar to have an invasive procedure done. They ask why their own dentist can't do the procedure, and why the dentist needs to refer. Some dentists may feel a bit defensive, perhaps little inadequate, though they know the benefits to the patient. They have a hard time expressing to the patient that the specialist is better trained, better equipped, faster and can provide greater safety and comfort. So they scare the contents out of the patient by overstating the situation: "The tooth is *wrapped around your nerve, and if I made a mistake your lip will drag on your shoe for the rest of your life!"* Or something like, "The tooth is in your sinus," or "I might break your jaw because the tooth is so deep in the weakest part of the jaw." This increases the patient anxiety unnecessarily, and it may lead to a general anesthesia where the surgeon may have been able to do an easy and comfortable procedure under local anesthesia.

Simply say, "I don't do that procedure as a matter of training and my practice design. You will receive excellent care by meeting with my OMS for consultation and treatment." Reassure the patient in ways that provide benefits for seeing your chosen specialist, without creating undue anxiety about the complexity or potential for complications. Leave that to the surgeon. They typically provide excellent informed consent procedures.

Emergency Procedures

Emergency procedures are another reason a general dentist may choose to refer a patient. You are a bit behind in a busy afternoon, and a patient calls with pain and swelling. Your harried patient coordinator comes to the operatory to tell you she needs guidance about how to "fit the patient into the schedule," (which is another story). You decide the best thing is to have the patient seen by a specialist as a matter of convenience.

This scenario is the cardinal sin of poor specialist relations. It is especially egregious if you are an infrequent referral source, or if this is the only type of circumstance in which you refer. Oral surgeons refer to this as patient "dumping," and the category includes other patients deemed undesirable for various, usually professionally or ethically incorrect reasons; for instance, a suspicion that they are HIV positive. This is one of the situations described earlier that creates long waiting times in the surgeon's office.

The correct protocol for emergency patients is to first see them in your office as soon as they can get there. You can quickly evaluate the patient and decide whether:

1. You will treat the immediate pain or swelling...
   A. to later refer to the appropriate specialist, or
   B. to later complete treatment yourself.
2. You will refer to an OMS.
3. You will refer to an endodontist.

If the telephone interview with the receptionists indicates, it *may be* appropriate to have the doctor talk to the patient to confirm the *need* for an immediate surgical referral. This really saves very little time, since the doctor will be required to do reasonably careful investigation, which is much more difficult over the phone. Depending upon the time of day, and the circumstances this may be the most practical solution to getting a true emergency patient into the surgeon's office as soon as possible.

These are situations where proper professional etiquette calls for a personal telephone contact by the doctor. This indicates to the surgeon and his or her staff that the patient is not being "dumped," and that you are personally involved and concerned. It communicates your practice philosophy is observed in all conditions, especially when inconvenient. Personally thanking the office staff and the surgeon for their prompt and helpful attention will greatly inspire a positive attitude toward your practice and your referrals.

Surgical procedures have a certain risk of post operative pain, infection and other complications. These are the surgeon's responsibilities, but the general dentist should be informed of any unhappy events. It is standard procedure among surgeons to call post-surgical patients in the evening after surgery. This should be a clear policy between you and your surgeon. The surgeon is responsible for the care and the follow-up, but you need to be in the loop of information. If there is a complication, the general dentist should be informed the next day. At that point, the general dentist should provide whatever support and patient communication the surgeon and general dentist mutually feel is appropriate. It is sometimes helpful if the general dentist makes one call to check in and reassure the patient and express confidence in the surgeon. The purpose of the call is not to assume any responsibility or to minimize the events, just to express concern and to reassure the patient. This is a policy matter between the doctors that must be discussed in advance, but psychologically it is a boost for the patient.

Think about what you can do to influence a positive outcome from the patient's point of view: Imagine you just had a surgical procedure done yesterday, and one of the complications you hoped would not happen, did happen. You are homebound or in the hospital, and either numb or in pain, swollen or otherwise incapacitated. Your surgeon has spoken to you once last night, and again today. You are feeling sorry you ever had the procedure done and are wondering why you ever decided to do it. You may even be wondering if something went wrong or wasn't done properly. You might be considering whom to sue. Then your general dentist calls, "just to check in to see how you're doing—I heard you have some concerns or questions." You then hear confirmation from your dentist who referred you that the procedure was necessary, that the unexpected does occur, that the doctors have seen this before and other reassuring comments. Your dentist expresses confidence in your surgeon. After the call, you definitely *feel* better.

Here, again, are some caveats: Do not do anything that contradicts the surgeon's decisions or explanations. He or she is responsible for the procedure and the outcome. If what you do or say can be construed as treatment, or as taking over of the case, you will assume full liability for the outcome. Do not visit the patient or see the patient in your practice; do not prescribe medications, take over treatment of a dry socket or change dressings without consultation and direction from the OMS. They will always do these things for the patient; they will not appreciate what is truly interference if you intervene in any way. Yet, this is not a fine line at all. It is simply common sense. Support your patient by supporting your surgeon.

Here are the steps to establish excellent communication with your oral and maxillofacial surgeon:

1. Visit several surgeons if possible, meet and discuss clinical philosophy.
2. Select a surgeon who most closely mirrors your philosophy.
3. If you are limited to a single surgeon or none in your area who closely mirrors your philosophy, then:
   A. Complete a *Practice Philosophy* and share it with your chosen surgeon.
   B. Ask for input from the surgeon on how you can align your practices to provide this level of care. Be sure to demonstrate benefits to the surgeon. Don't dwell on deficiencies, describe the positive environment and outcomes you hope to achieve.

   C. Take the surgeon's comments and edit and combine them into your *Practice Philosophy* so that it becomes a *Joint Statement of Philosophy.*

4. Develop referral forms and Standard Operating Procedures for referrals that reflect this mutual philosophy. Your surgeon will probably want to be the source of the actual forms and will provide them for you at no cost to you.
5. Implement the procedures and review the success or disappointment.

Here is a sample Standard Operating Procedure for Surgical Referrals:

REQUEST FOR SURGICAL CONSULTATION OR TREATMENT

[consult.10]

Desired Outcome: To have a patient receive specialized services from an oral and maxillofacial surgeon who will provide a successful surgical procedure with proficiency and compassion.

Measurement: The procedure is completed. The patient is satisfied and reports favorably on the experience of hospitality, clinical and administrative proficiency and follow-up.

1. Doctor diagnoses the need for a surgical treatment and documents it in the patient record. Decision is made to refer.
2. Assistants do not determine to whom the patient is referred.
3. The referral is formalized on **Request for Surgical Consultation or Treatment** form, filled out and signed by the doctor.
4. The form is an NCR triplicate. Mail or FAX the top copy to the surgeon, keep the second copy, and give the third copy to the patient. A copy of the form follows this SOP.
5. The receptionist or patient coordinator assists the patient with making an appointment with the surgeon's office according to mutually developed protocols.
6. Place the NCR form in doctor's "Telephone Return" message box. Doctor will call and briefly describe the referral with the surgeon during the next telephone message call period.

Request For Surgical Consultation or Treatment / 2

If the referral deviates from routine:

7. Doctor will indicate special circumstances on the referral slip.
8. Doctor will either write or dictate a referral letter to Dr. S detailing the specific circumstances of the referral. It is usually a good idea to include the patient's detailed medical history and treatment plan for exceptional referrals.
9. In cases of multiple specialties, special cases like cleft lip/palate, or challenging reconstruction or implant cases, a meeting between the doctors is indicated. Receptionist will arrange the meeting at the earliest mutual convenience.
10. Case planning and progress meetings will be held as necessary. Receptionist is to schedule those meetings upon verbal notice.
11. In necessary cases, after exam and prior to treatment, the surgeon will call to confirm the diagnosis and report on the scheduling for the procedure. Such calls are reason to interrupt the doctor.
12. The surgeon often will call after procedures to report surgical completion and any complications.
13. Doctor may follow-up with patient by phone one day after surgery. A telephone message will be prepared by the clinical coordinator and placed into doctor's "Telephone Return" message box on the proper day as a reminder.

EMERGENCY CONSULTATIONS

[emercons.10]

Desired Outcome: To have a patient receive specialized services from an oral surgeon or endodontist who will provide a successful specialty procedures with proficiency and compassion.

Measurement: The procedure is completed. The patient is free of pain and infection, is satisfied, and reports favorably on the experience of hospitality, clinical and administrative proficiency and follow-up.

1. Doctor diagnoses the need for an emergency treatment and documents it in the patient record. Decision is made to refer.
2. Assistants do not determine to whom the patient is referred.
3. The referral is formalized on either the **Surgical Referral** form, or the **Endodontic Referral** form, filled out and signed by the doctor.
4. The form is an NCR triplicate. FAX the top copy to the specialist, or give the top copy to the patient to take to the specialist. Keep the second copy, and give the third copy to the patient. A copy of the form follows this SOP.
5. The receptionist or patient coordinator assists the patient with making an appointment with the specialist's office according to mutually developed protocols.
6. Doctor will speak to the specialist doctor as soon as possible.

Emergency Consultations / 2

If the referral deviates from routine:

7. Doctor will indicate special circumstances on the referral slip.
8. Doctor will describe exceptional circumstances in an immediate telephone consultation.
9. The specialist may call to confirm the diagnosis and report on the procedure. Such calls are reason to interrupt the doctor.
10. Doctor may follow-up with patient by phone tomorrow. A phone message slip will be prepared by the clinical coordinator and placed into doctor's "Telephone Return" message box as a reminder.

SURGICAL REQUESTS

[surgreqs.10]

Introducing:

Patient's Name ________________________________ Date __________
Address ____________________ City ____________ State ____ ZIP _____
Telephone _____________ FAX _______________ E-mail ____________

Medical history:

Dental history and treatment plan:

Services requested; indicate teeth by description and location:

Indicate missing teeth with an "X," teeth to be extracted with a "/", implant sites with an "i":

1	2	3	4	5	6	7	8	9	10	11	12	13	14	15	16
32	31	30	29	28	27	26	25	24	23	22	21	20	19	18	17

Special circumstances or requests; other specialists involved:

☐ Referral letter to follow
☐ Case planning meeting requested

THANK YOU!

Signed ________________________________ D.D.S.

ENDODONTIC EMERGENCY REQUESTS

[endoreqs.10]

Introducing:

Patient's Name ______________________________ Date __________
Address ____________________ City ____________ State ____ ZIP _____
Telephone _____________ FAX ________________ E-mail _____________

Medical history:

Dental history and treatment plan:

Services requested; indicate teeth by description and location:

☐ Exam and report teeth underlined
☐ Treat teeth circled
☐ Exam and report non-specific or non-isolated pain:
☐ UR ☐ UL ☐ LL ☐ LR

Indicate missing teeth with an "X," circle teeth to be endodontically treated, underline teeth in question:

1	2	3	4	5	6	7	8	9	10	11	12	13	14	15	16
32	31	30	29	28	27	26	25	24	23	22	21	20	19	18	17

Special circumstances or requests; other specialists involved:

☐ Referral letter to follow

THANK YOU!

Signed ________________________________ D.D.S.

Chapter 11

THE BLACK TRIANGLE: PROBLEMS OF PERIODONTAL COMMUNICATION

"I stopped referring to periodontists a couple of months ago because I felt I was losing money and patients. My periodontist got all the expensive procedures, and the patients got lost in his practice." Steve said. "I even think he diverted some of them to another general dentist."

"How has your new policy worked out?" I inquired.

"Fairly well. We hired a consultant to help us "turbo charge" our hygiene department. We follow our own protocols for billing; we do all of our own root planing and surgical procedures," he reported.

"I am impressed!" I said. "The explosion in periodontal technology in the last few years has been enormous. How do you keep up with all the procedures and literature?" I asked.

"We took a course in laser surgery, and I had all my hygienists become laser certified. We almost have no surgery to do because our laser curettage and laser gingival surgeries provide such a complete result," he claimed.

"And are you profitable in this area?" I asked.

"I really don't know. That's why I hired you," Steve confessed. "I hop from chair to chair, and you know how out of control my overhead is..."

*　　　*　　　*

In the past four years, the ***Practice Operations Survey*** conducted by the Pankey Institute has proven that high volume hygiene practices are less profitable than well controlled hygiene practices. The intuitive decisions made by dentists and dental management companies that bigger is better simply does not hold true for hygiene. Economic and management journals continue to publish articles making these claims with no statistical proof.

Periodontal technology has advanced more rapidly than any specialty in recent years. Today it is possible to correct mucogingival defects, both by increasing the width of the attachment apparatus and creating esthetic root coverage, to create more favorable restorative environments, and even encourage regeneration of bone. The specificity of the various periodontal surgical procedures is quite precise. Periodontal prosthetic case planning and case results are far superior to where they were even two or three years ago, and new developments are reported monthly.

Enlightened periodontists have in their armamentarium techniques that can provide previously unimaginable results. If invited into the case planning process early, a periodontist can make suggestions for services that will provide for greater cleansibility, comfort, longevity and even esthetics. In simple cases, they can help solve vexing problems of short crowns and irregular gingival display from tooth migration or poorly performed orthodontics, and the esthetic challenges associated with the relationship of the smile line. Periodontists often have a better understanding of occlusion, restorative dentistry and tissue health maintenance than many oral surgeons, and therefore, are a valuable resource for implant treatment planning, surgical placement and maintenance in many communities.

Conversely, the trend in general practice over the last decade has been to de-emphasize the role of the periodontist in case planning. This is apparently the result of a shift in business concepts and certain management theories that create the expectation of higher profits from hygiene "departments." Once considered the "loss leader" of general practice, hygiene departments are now being created and pushed to become a major profit center, even the most significant profit center of practices with over-expanded hygiene production models. In the "*new hygiene*" paradigm, the hygienists are responsible for 30 to 40 percent or more of the total office production. Almost every major consulting company is advocating some form of this expanded hygiene model. Unfortunately, the model is based upon erroneous business assumptions that claim this expansion of hygiene programs will yield greater profits.

In reality, it's been more like the "Sorcerer's Apprentice" in many practices, with scheduling and accelerated activity getting completely out of hand. The expected "profit centers" have not proven to be as profitable as they are expansive of overhead. Evidence of this is available from studies conducted by the L.D. Pankey Institute Business Services Development Department, along with the Gallup Organization.[1] In these studies, the high hygiene producers were not found to be the most profitable practices. A more conservative model of quality practice where about 20 percent of the total office production is due to hygiene is also the most

[1] See *High Performance Hygiene: Overhauling Practice Economics;* Dental Practice & Finance, July/Aug., 1997, and the rebuttal by Richard Green, D.D.S., *High Performance Hygiene: a better model;* Dental Practice & Finance, Sept./Oct. 1997

profitable model. This, of course necessitates a dynamic and purposeful relationship with at least one periodontal practitioner to support the general dentist's need for specialty services.

Yet, misconceptions of what constitutes a model hygiene program abound. One hygiene presenter developed a model based upon accounting principles and applied it to an insurance model for dental practice. His assumptions are that more is better and expansion always brings greater profits. It appears to be an "easy money" scheme, but patient care gets lost in the mix. "Soft Tissue Management," under a variety of disguises including "Supportive Periodontal Therapy" or "SPT" (sounds like "spit") has become the financial cash cow, allowing the quality of patient care to easily slip. A careful analysis of how standards of periodontal care are determined in these practices shows an over-reliance on simple probing depth numbers. Little or no emphasis is placed on mucogingival problems, nor understanding issues such as the biological width and pre-prosthetic crown preparation, let alone beneficial elective esthetic procedures such as ridge augmentations and root coverage. In these practices, patients are almost always being told that their success or failure is largely a matter of personal oral hygiene, which may or may not be the case, and are placed on very strict administrative follow-up for recalls that may not be appropriate for every patient.

Unfortunately, this trend has led to a deteriorating relationship between periodontists and many general practitioners just at a time when periodontal science and clinical technology have achieved unexpected advancement. Self-serving business trends have effectively eliminated the periodontist from the restorative treatment planning team in many practices. Relegated to "rescuing" impossibly advanced treatment cases, or attempting to rehabilitate someone else's failures, many periodontists are returning to the general practitioner "completed" surgical patients with very disappointing results. General dentists who read about and view images of highly successful procedures in journals, wonder why their patients don't receive such gorgeous results, not ever conceding that they have seldom sent their periodontist a patient at the appropriate time for a predictable result. Instead, these operators prefer to proceed on a profitable restorative treatment plan. Negative periodontal consequences are "managed" by a combination of "soft tissue management" or "supportive periodontal therapy," and by officious hygienists blaming the patient. After all, it's covered by insurance, right?

On the other hand, general dental attitudes have been partly shaped by the attitudes and performance of periodontists. Most general dentists have experienced problems similar to Steve's, where the patient is referred back to the general dentist following periodontal surgery, and the esthetic results are miserable. Or, patient after patient is referred to a certain periodontal office, never to be seen again. The periodontist seems to have his or her own "supportive periodontal therapy" program going, and the patients never graduate. Some periodontists are very critical of restorative dentistry and can undermine the relationship between the patient and his or her general dentist with subtle statements and innuendo. Reports are common from general dentists of complex cases being referred (diverted, really) to a prosthodontist without counsel with the referring dentist.

General dentists believe they are the clinical coordinators or "quarterbacks" of patient care. Ideally, patients are referred to specialists for reasonably discreet services over a limited time frame. Then they are sent back to the referring dentist for continuing care. It is not unreasonable for the referring doctor to expect the specialist to follow some preplanned protocols. It is not a question of "who's in charge?" as it is a matter of excellent inter-professional communications.

Let's take a look at a successful periodontal referral. The two doctors involved may not see it the same way. The general dentist wants the problems to be solved; yet he wants the patient back in his office in as little time as possible, with all of the patient's insurance benefits remaining. On the other hand, the periodontist wants enough time to observe the patient's oral hygiene and tissue health, follow-up with post-operative tissue healing, perform "touch-up" surgery or mucogingival procedures, and see the patient for a few periodontal maintenance visits to help ensure periodontal stability. Many periodontists want to repeat previously accomplished root planing performed at the general dental office. (Don't they trust the generalist—or her hygienist?)

Success will be dictated by the ability to communicate both the *Practice Philosophy*, that is your *general expectations* that apply to all referred cases, and the specific needs of the case at hand. Your general expectations of hospitality, clinical proficiency, administrative proficiency, and follow-up should be established and confirmed prior to ever referring a single patient to *any* specialist's office. This is completed in a series of personal meetings with the periodontist. Then, the specific needs of the case at hand need to be communicated in a clear, concise and understandable fashion, so the periodontist knows what results you specifically seek for this patient. This is accomplished by a standard operating procedure for referrals that should include a standard referral slip and a referral letter. In very simple cases a letter may not be necessary. A telephone call will do. But don't be lulled into the typical standard of care where every case is treated casually and informally. Such a lax standard will result in unsuccessful patient and professional relationships. Ultimately, casual communications create a *casualty* of patient care, perhaps even a lawsuit that could have been avoided.

So it becomes critical to communicate treatment goals and expectations to the periodontist to maximize quality of patient care and treatment outcomes. One way to help establish communication is to determine the personality traits of the periodontist.

1. The **counselor**: This periodontist wants to spend time getting to know everything about the patient and concentrates in detail on his or her oral hygiene. She may hold the patient to an unrealistic standard for home care. She may repeat root planing sessions and tend to use up a lot of the patient's time. Furthermore, she never seems to get to definitive therapy, and if she does, it is followed by a long period of post-operative evaluation. Operating from a soft tissue management paradigm, this doctor's practice is definitely a "black triangle" where patients will disappear. In addition to all this grief, many times you may be able to do as well in your own practice without the need of referral.
2. The **perfectionist**: This guy was a really good technical operator in school, but couldn't get his crown and bridge truly *perfect.* This lead to frustration and later specialization in another area of dentistry. He tends to be hypercritical of other's restorative work and diverts patients to his chosen few dentists, often to a prosthodontist. This is another "black triangle," but in some ways worse, because you may be a member of his rogue's gallery and not know it.
3. The **surgeon**: This one likes to cut, and enjoys patients referred for a specific surgical procedure. If you have a clear treatment plan, know the surgical options available in the field and are able to bring your patients up to a pre-surgical standard, then this can be an excellent relationship. Maintenance may be a problem, since he may not be interested in an ongoing relationship with the patient or alternate recare visits.

4. The **architect**: Try to find one like this. This is a periodontist who likes challenges and knows the technology. She can assist you in the early stages of treatment planning, works cases up quickly, offers creative and clever solutions and gets to definitive therapy in a timely manner. She will coordinate schedules with you in order to have you present during certain surgeries to place final restorative margins. If she is really good, she'll place the final margin for you at your request during surgery to create an ideal margin that allows for biological width and cleansibility. She has an understanding of occlusion and restorative dentistry, and can develop a "big picture" approach which integrates periodontics, orthodontics and restorative dentistry.

Patient expectations are also important for successful referrals. Most patients do not like to be "referred out," and will question the need to involve another dentist. These objections are to be expected, and each one should be addressed to the patient's satisfaction. Once past the objections, a key element to success is to help shape the patient's expectations of the experience and the results. Periodontal treatment results, like all other facets of dentistry, should not be oversold. Periodontal procedures are useless without a comprehensive treatment plan. A single brick does not make a wall. The patient who is aware that this is a step toward the larger goal you have mutually identified will fare better emotionally with the interim results and post-operative sequelae. Keep the messages you want to convey to the patient simple, clear and consistent. Outline the benefits such as preservation of their teeth, longevity of the restorative dentistry, or ultimately the cosmetic result. Shape and frame the benefits in light of the goals you mutually agreed to during the formulation of your comprehensive treatment plan. Avoid spending time listing benefits you know do not concern a particular patient.

An enlightened periodontist to assist you with complex treatment planning and delivery of comprehensive dental care is an asset. Careful development of a loyal, dynamic and purposeful relationship with your periodontist will bring professional satisfaction and predictable clinical success.

Here are the steps to forming a high-value relationship with your periodontist:

1. Visit several periodontists to meet and discuss clinical philosophy.
2. Select a periodontist who most closely mirrors your philosophy.
3. Share your *Practice Philosophy* with the candidate.
4. If you are limited to a single periodontist, or none in your area, who closely mirror your philosophy, then:
   A. Complete a *Practice Philosophy,* and share it with your chosen periodontist.
   B. Ask for input from the periodontist on how you can align your practices to provide this level of care. Be sure to demonstrate benefits to the periodontist. Don't dwell on deficiencies; describe the positive environment and outcomes you hope to achieve.
   C. Take the periodontist's comments and edit and combine them into your *Practice Philosophy* so that it becomes a *Joint Statement of Philosophy.*
5. Develop referral forms and Standard Operating Procedures for referrals that reflect this mutual philosophy. There are samples of Standard Operating Procedures and Referral Slips below.
6. Implement the procedures.

PERIODONTAL REFERRALS

[perioref.11]

Desired Outcome: To have a patient receive specialized services from a periodontist who will provide successful periodontal therapies and surgical procedures with proficiency and compassion, expediently and with loyalty to this practice.

Measurement: Periodontal exam, treatment plan, and consultation with doctor is completed expediently. Therapies are completed efficiently and successfully. The patient is referred back to our practice. He is satisfied and reports favorably on the experience of hospitality, clinical and administrative proficiency and follow-up. We are able to proceed with the next phase of treatment.

1. Doctor diagnoses the need for a periodontal specialist evaluation and documents it in the patient record.
2. Assistants do not determine to whom the patient is referred.
3. The referral is formalized on the **Periodontal Referral** form, and signed by the doctor.
4. The form is an NCR triplicate. Mail or FAX the top copy to the periodontist, keep the second copy, and give the third copy to the patient. A copy of the form follows this SOP.
5. The receptionist or patient coordinator assists the patient in making an appointment with the periodontal office according to mutually developed protocols.

Periodontal Referrals / 2

6. Place the NCR form in doctor's "Telephone Return" message box. Doctor will call and discuss the patient with the periodontist during the next telephone message call period.
7. Doctor will indicate special circumstances on the referral slip.
8. Doctor will either write or dictate a referral letter to the periodontist detailing the specific circumstances of the referral, the patient's initial treatment plan and ultimate goals, the patient's detailed medical history, and goals of periodontal therapy.
9. In cases of multiple specialties or challenging reconstruction or implant cases, a meeting between the doctors is indicated. Receptionist will arrange the meeting at the earliest mutual convenience.
10. Case planning and progress meetings will be held as necessary. Receptionist is to schedule those meetings upon verbal notice.
11. In all cases, after exam and prior to treatment, the periodontist is expected to call and to confirm the diagnosis and report on the scheduling for the procedure. Such calls are reason to interrupt the doctor, who may need to be present for certain procedures.
12. The periodontist is expected to call and/or write a letter after procedures to report of surgical completion and any complications.
13. Doctor will follow-up with patient by phone one day after any periodontal surgeries. A telephone message will be prepared by the patient coordinator and placed into doctor's "Telephone Return" message box on the proper day as a reminder.

PERIODONTAL REFERRAL SLIP

[perioref.11]

Introducing:

Patient's Name ______________________________ Date ________
Address __________________ City __________ State ___ ZIP ____
Telephone ____________ FAX _____________ E-mail ___________

Medical history:

Dental history and treatment plan:

- ☐ See attached comprehensive treatment plan
- ☐ Root planing completed on ____________
- ☐ No root planing to date
- ☐ Patient currently on _______ month recare interval
- ☐ Prefer alternate recare
- ☐ Maintenance in our office only

Services requested; indicate teeth by description and location:

Indicate missing teeth with an "X," circle expected surgical sites, indicate implant sites with an "i":

1	2	3	4	5	6	7	8	9	10	11	12	13	14	15	16
32	31	30	29	28	27	26	25	24	23	22	21	20	19	18	17

Special circumstances or requests; other specialists involved:

☐ Radiographs forwarded ☐ Patient to deliver radiographs
☐ Please order radiographs ☐ Referral letter to follow
☐ Case planning meeting requested

THANK YOU!

Signed ________________________________ D.D.S.

Chapter 12

BANDING TOGETHER: SOLVING ORTHODONTIC PROBLEMS

An innovation of dental management and marketing—the publicly owned orthodontic practice—has appeared on the scene in several major urban markets. Publicly held corporations are widely accepted and embraced in the consumer economy. This business structure allows the public to share in the profits of the organization and creates opportunities for investors—large and small—to participate in the national and global economies. Public ownership of corporations motivated solely by profit is a valuable and honored economic reality. It is also completely repugnant to professional ethics.

Professionals, whether lawyers, physicians or dentists all share the ethical duty of placing their clients' welfare before their own. One of the basic tenets of a professional is the ability to govern one's own actions and professional organization. One of the protections the public has *previously* enjoyed is the prohibition against anyone other than a professional owning a professional practice. Today, we see these proscriptions breaking down and professionalism is being lost in the corporate structure of today's "professional" marketplace. Physicians are now largely employed by HMOs or working entirely for insurance organizations. Federal anti-trust actions have lowered or eliminated any barriers against most forms of advertising. Now we see overtly misleading ads officially ignored because the bureaucratic definition of consumer rights is tipped toward price reduction as the greatest public benefit.

Yet there is a dark side even for these pioneers of professional collapse. Medical managed care organizations, once the sweetheart of Wall Street, are now becoming embroiled in costly fraud and anti-trust litigation as well as consumer tort actions in medical malpractice. Physicians are now feeling the economic pressure of poor economic decisions. HMOs have apparently extracted all the potential savings from a once bloated medical care system, and now consumers are going to again see medical costs rise far in excess of the national economic inflation.

So the time seems right for a sojourn by profiteers into publicly held dental corporations. Professional ethics will be low on the corporate priority for these groups. Expect professional practice standards to be equally ignored. When an organization is chartered for the purpose of quarterly profits for investors, they have control over the decisions the employees make. This is clearly a conflict of interest for the dentist-employees who choose to practice in such an environment and will be told how to practice. Criteria for diagnosis, treatment planning and treatment timing will be corporate decisions. Patient care will have the commodity-based feel of any other corporate factory, and patients will be considered units of production, there for potential profit.

Dentists need to be aware of two major elements of this trend. The first is that these practices market to the public directly and bypass the general dentist. The kind of dynamic communication and professional influence that we are advocating in this philosophy will be impossible if your patients are lured into these practices. The second element is these practices will market themselves in ways that are very visible in the community. This will put pressure on the general dentist to identify and communicate benefits to the patient to seek the services of a quality orthodontic practice. This must be done in a positive way, discussing the patient's personal needs and the benefits of a coordinated treatment plan. Making negative or disparaging comments about the corporate orthodontic office to patients will harm the profession and your relationship with patients. The public will be very aware of the low price offered in these clinics, and eventually everyone will know someone who has been treated there. Like the large HMO dental clinics, these corporate orthodontic offices will provide the pinnacle of hospitality and consumer orientated quality features such as location, parking, landscaping, architecture and surroundings and a pleasant, well-groomed staff. The prices will be low, the payment plans simple.

Orthodontic offices will be forced to respond to this phenomenon. In fact, all orthodontic practices are subject to the same economic pressure that inspired the creation of the corporate practice. The emergence of these clinics is the result of some universal changes in the management of all orthodontic practices. Most orthodontic practices now report as much as 50 percent of their new patients are referrals from their past and present patients. The general dentist, if the patient has one, is identified and consulted after the initial patient contact, in many cases after treatment is initiated. The trend is each year more newcomers are patient-referred, and fewer referrals are from general dentists. Many orthodontists have come to the inevitable conclusion that they need to market not only to their referring dentists, but must also have a patient-based internal marketing program. Some are introducing direct external marketing to the public, especially in areas of high professional saturation and incursion of corporate practices.

Another pressure is price competition, coupled with the lack of sophistication or discernment of the public regarding different levels of orthodontic care and service. Advertising price competition has been considered an ethical breach by professionals in the past. In well founded ethical systems, professional pricing is grounded in *fairness* to the patient and to the doctor. Fees are determined *individually* after all the factors of a particular case are weighed. Factors that may be considered are the complexity of the case, special skills or training involved, the length of time it will take, special requirements the patient may have, or special difficulties or challenges the patient creates and the patient's ability to pay. Some cases bring a high professional fee. Others are done for nothing, hopefully by the doctor's choice and not because of poor financial arrangements. The least important factor should be price-centered marketing from competitors.

Yet the commodity-minded orientation of today's insurance culture has left professional ethics behind. Today price competition may be the greatest pressure your orthodontist feels. Remember that point as we move on with the rest of this discussion. You may conclude that it is impossible for an orthodontist to fulfill his obligations to your *Practice Philosophy* if he or she is mainly focused on profits and on public external marketing. Your practice is incidental to this doctor. If orthodontists overreact to these new competitive pressures, the ultimate result may be that none are distinguishable from the other. The challenge for the general dentist who has patient-centered care in mind will be to maintain a dynamic relationship with an equally patient-centered orthodontist who will provide a quality service for his or her patients.

Orthodontic services are needed by about 70 percent of the population. In other words, that percentage of people *could benefit* from some level of orthodontic therapy. Each patient seen by a qualified general dentist is evaluated for occlusal problems, some of which will require orthodontic treatment. Patients committed to orthodontic treatment establish a long-term relationship with another office, which becomes in many instances their only dental interface for many months, even years. Here is where the communication link is so essential in preserving the patient's relationship with your practice and to commencing comprehensive restorative care as soon as possible.

The first step is to encourage the patient to see an ethical, patient-centered orthodontist with whom you share a *Practice Philosophy.* When the need for orthodontic services is identified, the patient may be led to your preferred outcome by making statements of *benefits* that fit the patient's previously identified goals. Once the patient is receptive to referral to your chosen orthodontist, the *features* of the therapy and your clinical goals can be clearly and simply presented. Get patient commitment *first,* then move on to the details.

Incorporating orthodontic therapy in the treatment planning of adolescents is relatively straightforward. In most adolescents, orthodontia is probably the greatest single dental need, and the general dental or comprehensive restorative treatment plan is usually very basic. Adults, which comprise an ever-increasing percentage of orthodontic cases, usually have a much more involved comprehensive treatment plan. Orthodontic therapy usually falls quite early in the development of a reconstruction case, after initial periodontal therapy and restorative provisionalization. Once the patient has entered treatment with the orthodontist, continued contact with your office is essential for long term patient relations, compliance with periodontal therapy and oral hygiene regimens and continued enthusiasm for the comprehensive treatment plan.

Orthodontists experience different challenges from different patient profiles. In general, the best adult orthodontic patients are those who have discussed the need for orthodontics with their general dentist and received a referral for treatment. On the other hand, the worst patients are those who initiated treatment for purely cosmetic reasons and decided to enter the practice on their own. Like "cosmetic dentistry," which some dentists now oversell, creating unrealistic expectations for results and durability, "cosmetic orthodontics" as understood by the uninformed patient brings high expectations with little understanding of limitations. These problems may become the bane of dentists in the near future. Dentistry and orthodontics have become too casual about elective procedures, which are becoming oversold in most egregious ways. It is too easy to begin treatment without proper planning or consultation, and misinformed and disappointed patients are the all too common result. In all forms of practice, there is pressure to find "profit centers" and to increase volume rather than to increase the quality of care and patient service. The result is an increase in patient expectations coupled with a reduction in appreciation for the art and science of the profession—a very dangerous combination. What used to be a mysteriously technical, artistic and almost miraculous transformation—either restoratively or orthodontically—is now merely "hip." There is a clear correlation between the reduction of fees in lower quality practices and the lowering of public perceptions and appreciation of dental and orthodontic care.

As a general rule, orthodontic patients should be seen for prophy and examination about every three months in the general dental office. When the two practices involved are well run and communicate with each other, these appointments can be coordinated so the arch wire is first removed by the orthodontic team, and the patient then presents for exam and prophy. This allows for periodic imaging, and better access for instrumentation and visual examination. Periodic vertical bitewings and periapicals on adult patients are a prudent policy. Consider this benefit when you analyze the geographic location of the orthodontist you choose. Of course, the ideal is to have all your specialists grouped around you in the same building or even the same office.

Professional communications with your orthodontist are essential for proper orthodontic results. Certainly no complex restorative case can be completed independently by even the most skilled orthodontist. The orthodontist needs to have a summary of your comprehensive treatment plan and ultimate treatment goals. It should also be established in the pretreatment consultation which dentist will plan and execute the equilibration, which is a required final step in nearly all orthodontic cases. Establishing effective orthodontic communications involves four stages, initial referral, pretreatment consultation, ongoing therapeutic consultation (case in progress) and case completion.

Initial referral is discussed above. Here the goal is really very simple: successfully directing the patient to your chosen orthodontist. Once the patient has committed to your chosen orthodontist, your confidence in the outcome is now very high. A **Standard Operating Procedure** for orthodontic referrals and **Orthodontic Referral Slip** are included at the end of this chapter.

The pretreatment consultation is best if the doctors personally meet. The restorative dentist can bring his or her models and other records and the orthodontist provides his or hers as well. The comprehensive treatment plan is reviewed and ultimate goals of treatment are discussed. Then the goals of orthodontic treatment are explored, with consideration of the benefits to the end results desired.

In a vacuum, the orthodontic case may progress and end very differently than without this important interface. For example, consider a Class II Division 2 case in an adult. Treatment options may include orthognathic surgery, extraction of premolar teeth or other approaches. What if the general dentist had completed a case mock-up on study models that included a trial equilibration and composite trial restorations on the anterior teeth, demonstrating excellent anterior guidance that indicates the case may be successfully treated without surgery? This should influence the orthodontist's decision, effectively simplifying the case, since the team approach allows him to rely on the comprehensive nature of the treatment plan to bring the case to a completed, ideal occlusion. He no longer has to present the more invasive surgical approaches to the patient and can provide superb service personally tailored to the particular needs of this patient. Just as likely, the case evaluations may prove the need for surgery, and the patient can then be given consistent, non-conflicting advice from the two doctors.

Once the case is underway, the orthodontist sees the patient monthly, and the general dentist sees the patient about every three months. (It is a good policy for the doctors to have quarterly visits with each other, usually over a light lunch, where they review the records and progress of all shared cases under treatment.) That afternoon, write a brief note to the patient to let him know of the meeting, and include any encouraging comments you can think of regarding his treatment. This establishes a link between the patient and the two practices, letting the patient know the quality and level of professional involvement he is getting. It also goes a long way to provide for patient goodwill and internal marketing. As the case nears completion, it is important that the general dentist reviews progress models and carefully examines the patient to assure the desired goals have been achieved. This must be confirmed with the orthodontist at a quarterly meeting.

Finally, the day the braces are removed should never be ignored by the general dental office. Most patients are anxious to have this day arrive, and it is an exciting time in his or her life. The orthodontist's patient coordinator must communicate *without fail* the dates of appliance removal. This allows you to schedule an afternoon or next-day early morning prophy and fluoride treatment and provide the patient with a small celebration. Simply come in and examine the patient, comment favorably on a job well done, and present the patient with a token gift such as a coffee mug or a single flower. This is not only a great marketing event, but it welcomes the patient back to your office and provides a simple rite of passage to the next stage of the treatment plan. This simple gesture helps you maintain the emotional involvement and commitment of the patient and keeps the momentum of treatment moving forward.

ORTHODONTIC COMMUNICATIONS

[orthocom.12]

Desired Outcome: Successful orthodontic treatment from case identification and referral to case completion. Patient will remain a patient of this practice, not lose ground periodontally and ultimately proceed to completion of the comprehensive treatment plan.

Measurement: 90 percent of cases referred accept treatment recommendations; 100 percent of cases initiated go to completion; 100 percent return to this practice for comprehensive care.

1. Case is identified by doctor as an orthodontic referral.
2. Study models, images, and the patient record are provided for doctor to complete case study.
3. Comprehensive diagnosis and treatment planning are completed.
4. Consultation is scheduled by patient coordinator with the patient: to discuss and present benefits of orthodontic referral.
5. **Orthodontic Referral Slip** is completed and signed by the doctor.
6. Patient Coordinator places a telephone message in doctor's Telephone Return box to remind doctor to call the orthodontist.
7. Doctor will call the orthodontist for a brief patient introduction.
8. Patient coordinator assists the patient in making an exam appointment at the office of the chosen orthodontist.
9. Patient coordinator schedules a pretreatment consultation between the doctors.

Orthodontic Communications / 2

10. After orthodontic examination, the doctors meet at the pretreatment consultation to discuss and finalize the treatment plan.
    a. Patient coordinator places all records on doctor's desk for review the day before the pretreatment consultation.
    b. Doctor reviews the records, completes wax-up or mock-up and model equilibration if not done previously.
11. At all times during orthodontic treatment, the patient coordinator will include this patient's records in those assembled for quarterly consultations. Patient coordinator will schedule those meetings to be held over a light lunch or immediately at day's end.
12. Doctor will meet quarterly with the orthodontist to discuss all mutual cases in progress.
13. All orthodontic cases will be seen every three months by the hygienist and examined briefly by the doctor.
14. Patient coordinator will track all cases in progress and note cases nearing completion on the Orthodontic Patient Monitor. Notify the doctor so that a more complete occlusal examination can be scheduled when the case is nearing completion. Report this during the morning huddle.
15. Patient coordinator will coordinate the band removal date to allow for case completion celebration and prophy.
16. Patient coordinator is responsible for selecting a small gift and organizing a brief "recognition" or "celebration" for the patient on braces removal day.
17. Doctor will send a small thank you note to the orthodontist in response to his case completion letter.

ORTHODONTIC REFERRAL SLIP

[orthoref.12]

Introducing:

Patient's Name ______________________________ Date __________
Address ____________________ City ____________ State ____ ZIP _____
Telephone _____________ FAX _______________ E-mail ____________

Medical history:

Dental history and treatment plan:

☐ See attached comprehensive treatment plan
☐ Comprehensive treatment plan to follow

Services requested; indicate teeth by description and location:

Special circumstances or requests; other specialists involved:

☐ Referral letter to follow
☐ Case planning meeting requested

THANK YOU!

Signed __________________________________ D.D.S.

SAMPLE REFERRAL LETTER

[sampref.12]

JAY M. HISLOP, D.D.S.

Excellence in Dentistry

Gerry Bowman, D.D.S.
2231 Amber Drive
Stockton, CA 95299

Dear Gerry:

SUBJECT: RHONDA DONNER

This letter is to introduce Rhonda Donner to your practice. Rhonda is a 41-year-old female who presented to our office for initial examination with the following:

- Class II, Div. 2 Malocclusion, with a relatively straight and esthetically acceptable profile

- Moderate periodontitis

- Numerous broken down alloy and direct composite restorations

- Signs of wear and occlusal breakdown including cervical abfractions, posterior wear facets and anterior crossover facets.

- Symptoms of TMD including the following: Trigger point pain, headaches, limitation upon opening, bilateral early reciprocal clicks, a 1mm slide CO-CR. Please refer to occlusal exam record enclosed.

(Gerry Bowman, DDS, p. 2)

• Her goals for treatment are to look beautiful and feel more comfortable. She is a very attractive woman, but her worn anteriors and visibly darkened restorative work are cosmetic problems that definitely detract from her appearance. She is frustrated that no dentist has ever resolved these problems satisfactorily, and she cannot do anything about them herself.

• She has expressed to Judy, our patient coordinator, that this is a high priority at this time in her life. She has presented no barriers to treatment, other than some minor scheduling requests.

We have completed our exam and initial therapy which included:

• Referral to Dr. Ron Gordan for periodontal evaluation and therapy. Rhonda received initial periodontal therapy and mucogingival surgery with grafts in three quadrants. Final periodontal report from Dr. Gordan is enclosed.

• Occlusal therapy and TMJ stabilization with splint therapy. Rhonda is now comfortable and stable with a predictably reproducible centric relation. I have not equilibrated her mouth, anticipating definitive orthodontic therapy.

• Teeth # 3, 4, 8, 9, 11, 14, 15, 18, 19, 27, 29, 30, 31 have provisional crowns. These are lab processed acrylic, cemented with a permanent type cement and will remain stable for the duration of orthodontic therapy.

(Gerry Bowman, DDS, p. 3)

Our anticipated comprehensive treatment plan is:

1. Complete Orthodontic therapy to provide a result similar to that obtained on my model study, if possible.
2. Equilibrate to finalize the occlusal relationships.
3. New porcelain veneer restorations on 5, 6, 7, 8, 9, 10,11, 12, 13. Complete plan for anterior guidance.
4. Porcelain or porcelain fused to metal crowns on 18, 19, 20, 28, 29, 30, 31.
5. Porcelain or PFM crowns on 3, 4, 14, 15.

Would you please examine Rhonda and have Christine make arrangements with Lisa for our pre-treatment consultation. As always, we would like to coordinate visits for prophy and exam at least twice a year, though we will see Rhonda every three months for prophy.

We will plan on our normal protocol of quarterly case review consultations.

Thanks for your help with this interesting and challenging case.

Sincerely,

Jay M. Hislop, D.D.S.

JH:ct

Chapter 13

THE PATIENT IN PAIN: ENDODONTIC REFERRALS AND FOLLOW-UP

You know the scenario! It is about 2:20 in the afternoon and you are completing the adjustments for a final cementation of a complex restorative case. You have been looking forward to the delivery of this fine restoration, and expecting a beautiful and functionally perfect result. In the morning huddle, your patient coordinator had communicated the times during the day when it would be possible to see an emergency, and since there were no calls, you are now focused on the few remaining tasks of a very successful day. Then the call comes in—a patient in pain.

Your day has now taken on a new character. What was once the careful performance of a well written and properly rehearsed symphony of clinical and administrative music, now has the potential to deteriorate into the confusion and discord of a second-rate musician. Your carefully orchestrated plan could degenerate into chaos, or it could be a minor inconvenience handled quite simply, like a single broken string on a third row violin.

If your practice has excellent communications standards in place, these cases really have a simple decision tree.

1. First, in a quality practice, the doctor wants to examine the patient, even if just briefly. There are exceptions to this rule. For example, the endodontist is geographically distant from your office and near the patient. In that case the doctor may simply want to interview the patient on the phone, confirming the nature of the complaint is appropriate for immediate referral. The later in the day the emergency call comes in, the more likely it will be to follow this protocol. This is not simply for your convenience, but for the convenience of the endodontist and staff, and it serves the patient better and more efficiently as well. Nobody likes to be delayed from the planned events of his or her day, and even in a business such as ours, which can be filled with unexpected events, it is important to plan and organize in such a way that most days can proceed in a smooth and systematic manner. Look at the clock, and consider what one extra step may do to cause delay for the doctors and the patient who is in pain. Then make the decision that is in the best interest of the patient. But in most cases, the patient should be told to come to the office immediately. In many offices this can be done without disturbing the doctor.
2. The patient arrives and is seen briefly by the doctor.
3. A decision is made to treat or to refer. This decision is based upon several factors: (a) the clinical criteria the doctor uses to choose when endo will be treated in the practice, or referred; (b) the time available for the doctor to begin treatment; (c) the time of day; and (d) the patient's location.
4. If the patient is to be treated, the treatment is begun as soon as possible fitting the visit around other patient visits, following the office SOP for endodontic emergencies.

5. If the patient is to be referred, the endodontist is called immediately.

In some offices, the protocol becomes very simple, because the general dentists do no endodontics. In such a practice, the patient should be interviewed on telephone by the doctor, as soon as possible from the initiating call. The doctor needs to take or return this call to ascertain the patient symptoms and decide the appropriate referral. If the doctor needs to return the call, time is of the essence. The patient is in pain, and every minute is important to him or her. Imagine the first few minutes after a patient calls and is told the doctor will return the call as soon as possible. In most procedures, the doctor can break away after notice of an emergency call in from 1 to 15 minutes without causing any negative consequences to the current patient in the operatory. To the patient in pain who is waiting for a call, it feels like an hour or more. In a morning call, the return call must be made before lunch. If the call is not returned prior to a normal lunch hour, the patient will assume the doctor forgot and went to lunch, leaving the patient waiting in pain. If the call has not yet come in immediately after lunch, the patient will soon be looking for a new dentist.

So make the calls as soon as you can. It provides excellent patient care, improves the likelihood of a positive outcome, and tells the patient you really care about him or her—generating excellent good will and patient-based marketing for you.

Endodontists organize their practices to accommodate the emergencies from dozens of general, surgical, periodontal and prosthodontic practices. They accomplish their mission extremely well. The endodontist will see a patient, usually immediately, upon the referral from another doctor. Almost always, endodontists have 24 hour emergency call procedures arranged so that even the late day and after hours calls can be accommodated. It is a fabulous service to patients and to the referring doctors.

Yet this service can be easily taken for granted, and often abused. Many general practitioners have a desire to practice a wide range of services and endodontics is often in that mix. New technology, instruments and procedures are making the practice of endodontics easier, more predictable and more enjoyable. The new continuing education approaches are marvelous. So endodontic procedures have become more common, and more likely to be performed in the general practice. Some doctors have interpreted this to mean they no longer need to maintain an excellent working relationship with their endodontist.

The endodontist, on the other hand, has been challenged by the new technologies. Crown down preparation, canal "system" preparation, non-surgical retreatment, and warm gutta percha down-pack, back-pack fill techniques have created a new standard of care, raising the bar for the daily clinical results in the endodontic office. Mastery of new technology has been a major goal of most progressive endodontists in recent years. Patients have benefited from more predictable, long term results. General dentists need to keep all of this in mind when they choose to eliminate a quality endodontist from their team of specialists. The high level of service and excellent clinical results available from endodontic specialists make them a valuable member of any dental team.

When a general practitioner who has seldom or never referred to an endodontist finds a particularly recalcitrant case, the temptation is to declare it "impossible," and offer a "more predictable result" of extraction and prosthetics or implant. For a while in the early 1990s, it appeared that implants would soon usurp the need for any complicated or less predictable endodontic procedures. Why not just extract the tooth, preserving the maximum bone, and later place a cylinder implant? It seemed to be a prudent and effective protocol.

But endodontics rose to the challenge. Arguing that a tooth root, even endodontically treated is a more biologically acceptable entity than an implant, the research soon provided new ways to treat even the most complex teeth. Today the question remains unanswered. But for most cases, the option of root canal therapy, carefully completed using the most progressive measures, must be offered as a possible treatment plan in even the most difficult cases. Every general practitioner needs to have a place for his or her patients to receive such care.

The matter of patient scheduling and convenience is not trivial either. Today everyone is busy. The patient in pain has often interrupted very important activities and needs to get back on schedule. There is enormous pressure on patient coordinators to fulfill all the time demands made by patients. The doctor's schedule is carefully planned each day, usually with crossed fingers by the coordinator in hopes that no emergency call is received. When the call comes in, it often causes anxiety for everyone in the practice. A high standard of care in patient management really indicates that if your practice is not as well equipped to handle the emergency in as timely and efficient a manner as the specialist's office, then it really becomes your duty to offer the patient the option of a referral.

If you have not been referring patients on a reasonably regular basis, chances are you have poor or non-existent procedures for communication with an endodontist. This is a dangerous position to be in from a liability risk management perspective. If you are forced to take on clinical tasks that you cannot complete with the same standard of care as your local specialist, then you have little defense if the procedure fails to provide the expected result. The answer is simple. Be selective, and treat the endo you are comfortable with and for which you planned. But share the emergencies, and refer some interesting and challenging cases as well. Give you and your staff a break. The endodontist lives for your referrals, but if you abuse the emergency process, and only send him the impossible retreatments and difficult emergencies, it creates ill will and poor communication. Send him or her a routine case once in a while. Perhaps to create a chance to communicate, or to establish a positive balance in the good will account in that practice. It will pay off enormously when the most challenging emergency root canal problem arrives in your office on a late Friday evening.

Follow-up is the key to patient satisfaction in endodontic referrals. Courtesy and communication benefits dictate that the endodontist calls the referring dentist as soon as practical after examining the patient. If the referring doctor has not specified treatment, this call becomes mandatory, because the referring doctor has needed information about the comprehensive treatment plan that will usually influence endodontic treatment decisions. The tooth in question may have a guarded periodontal prognosis that would influence choices of treatment, for example.

After the doctors and the patient agree to treatment, and it is decided that the patient remain in the specialty practice for treatment, some foolproof follow-up procedures are needed to track the patient's care. This is best handled by tracking procedures in the endodontist's office, with a backup tickler system in the referring doctor's office. The endodontist may complete the treatment according to the patient's schedule, then inform the referring doctor of the case completion and document with appropriate images. On the referring side, a tracking system that creates a follow-up tickler to provide a reminder to check up on the patient is essential for clinical efficiency. If the referring doctor is in the midst of a restorative treatment, it is essential that this not be delayed longer than necessary. This is the **Endodontic Patient Monitor.** It is a three-part system that can be done by computer or by hand. Part one is the record of the patient visit and referral in the patient record. Part two is the posting on a monitor page of the date of referral, the doctor to whom the patient was referred, and the reason for referral. This can be a three ring binder monitor or a page in a computer management program. The third part is a card in a tickler file or a dated note in the computer that calls attention to the patient referral as a reminder to follow-up. The date of this depends upon the expected schedule for the patient, and the planned restorative treatment. It may be from two weeks to two months or more. When the reminder comes up, the chart is checked to see if the patient has returned to the office. If not, the specialist is called to determine the stage of treatment. The patient is then contacted for continued care or the tickler is reset for a later date, depending upon the circumstances of the treatment in the endodontist's office.

ENDODONTIC COMMUNICATIONS

[endocom.13]

Desired Outcome: Successful endodontic treatment from case identification and referral to case completion.

Measurement: Patient will be free of pain as rapidly as clinically possible, with no undue interruptions due to administrative practices. He or she will ultimately proceed to completion of the comprehensive treatment plan.

1. Patient presents in office as an emergency, and/or doctor identifies patient as having an endodontic problem requiring referral.
2. Images and diagnostic records are taken as needed.
3. Initial diagnosis and treatment plan are completed.
4. Patient coordinator consults with the patient to present and discuss benefits of endodontic referral. Often when a patient is in pain, the discussion is very simple. For more complex needs where the patient is not in pain, the doctor should complete a brief consultation and treatment plan presentation before sending the patient to the coordinator.
5. **Endodontic Referral Slip** is completed and signed by the doctor.
6. Doctor will call the endodontist for a brief patient introduction. If doctor cannot call immediately, patient coordinator places a telephone message in doctor's Telephone Return box to remind doctor to call the endodontist.
7. Patient coordinator assists the patient in making an exam appointment at the office of the chosen endodontist.
8. Patient coordinator will track all cases in progress and note cases nearing completion on the Endodontic Patient Monitor.

ENDODONTIC REFERRAL SLIP

[endoref.13]

Introducing:

Patient's Name ______________________________ Date _________
Address __________________ City ___________ State ___ ZIP ____
Telephone ____________ FAX ______________ E-mail ____________

Medical history:

Dental history and treatment plan:

Services requested; indicate teeth by description and location:

☐ Exam and report teeth underlined
☐ Treat teeth circled
☐ Exam and report non-specific or non-isolated pain:
☐ UR ☐ UL ☐ LL ☐ LR

Indicate missing teeth with an "X," circle teeth to be endodontically treated, underline teeth in question:

1	2	3	4	5	6	7	8	9	10	11	12	13	14	15	16
32	31	30	29	28	27	26	25	24	23	22	21	20	19	18	17

Special circumstances or requests; other specialists involved:

☐ Referral letter to follow

THANK YOU!

Signed ________________________________ D.D.S.

Chapter 14

ELMO GOES TO THE DENTIST: PEDIATRIC PRACTICE AND REFERRALS

Family dentistry is practiced by about 90 percent of all general practitioners. These dentists take care of nearly all the patients who walk or roll into their offices, any age, any disability. It is part of the life of the family dentist to be a generalist and to try to find solutions to care for as many patients as possible. Children represent some of the greatest joys and toughest challenges of family practice. Pediatric dentists cannot possibly take care of all the dental needs of children. In the State of California, for example, there are only about 350 pediatric dental specialists and about 17 million children. No matter how we do the math, there is no way for even a minority of general dentists to refer most or all of the children in their practice to a pediatric dentist. Fortunately during dental visits, most children exhibit reasonably predictable behaviors that fall well within the training and expertise of most general practitioners. But there are those few children who do not behave in predictable and manageable ways.

When a child is unable to adapt to the stresses of dental care, the general dentist has several options. There are of course many pressures to keep a patient in your own practice. The parents may have strong personal reasons or desires to keep the family in a single practice. Often these reasons are emotional or even sentimental, but have little rational basis. You may have financial incentives or penalties if you have agreements with the patient's insurance company. This is a purely economic reason, and if it leads to a decision that is against your professional judgment and counter to the standard of care, then you have breached an ethical and possibly legal duty. On the other hand, you may enjoy doing dentistry or orthodontics on slightly older patients, and hope to "get the child through" this early difficult stage.

You may have a professional interest in the care of children and dedicate substantial resources to continuing education for you and your staff in this area. Your expertise may be as good or better than any local pediatric dentist, and you may even be the happy recipient of children referred from other general dentists. Your practice may be geographically distant or inaccessible to a pediatric dentist, or the local one is unacceptable to you. In any case, you may have powerful professional incentives to learn to treat most of the patients in your practice. However, there are exceptions, and every dentist must be vigilant to the dangers that lurk in continued treatment of the behaviorally, medically or developmentally-compromised patient. The little patient that refuses or is unable to cooperate and becomes a "behavior management problem" can also quickly become a "risk management" problem. As the behavior problem becomes a barrier to proper treatment, the dentist must escalate his or her behavior management in ways that exert either physical or chemical control over the young patient. Then the dangers escalate as well.

In the broad view of a successful quality dental practice, careful application of certain communication techniques to control pediatric behavior should be the pre-determined policy of the doctor. If the patient can be managed by simple communication and behavior modification strategies, then they are an appropriate candidate for continued care in the family practice setting. If the patient does not respond to safe and conservative management, predictably and routinely, I recommend referral before *any* attempts are made to physically or chemically manage the patient, unless this is an area in which you have extensive training, *and* you perform the procedures routinely.

Otherwise, it is important to emphasize referral is ideally made prior to *any* restorative attempts. A decision must be made whether to escalate or to refer before control of the clinical situation is lost. This will, of course, tend to tilt the decision tree toward referral, but in today's perilous legal environment it is better to be safe than sorry. It is not only your patient's life, but the ongoing success of your practice that is at stake. Notice that this will still result in only a small percentage of all the pediatric patients in the practice being referred. In a survey of my own patients after 15 years of general practice, nearly 70 percent of all the children had only preventive and orthodontic services. Even if we referred *all* of the restorative cases, we would still have had a very successful family practice by any measure. Yet we were able to treat most of the restorative needs as well using only conservative behavior management techniques.

Very little restorative need exists in a well-managed population of pediatric patients who have excellent preventive care and fluoride. The restorative procedures can also be quite minimal; conservative air-abrasion procedures and sealants are the typical extent. In a quality practice, the need for advanced restorative procedures on children is so rare, that it is another criterion for referral.

Pediatric dentists have training to deal with behavioral problems in ways that are beyond the scope of most general dentists. They are also more effective if the child has not previously had a negative experience in a dental office. So the policy of the general dentist should be to evaluate and decide on treatment or referral before the treatment escalates to procedures that are unpredictable in the generalist's hands.

Referring a child to a pediatric dentist after several escalating and unsuccessful attempts to manage the child is an abuse of both the child and your relationship with the pediatric dentist. Such attempts reflect poorly on the competence of the general dentist—you, in this case—and create a handicap over which the pediatric dentist must then work hard to overcome, sometimes for many years. Both physical and psychological injury can occur in children when measures intended to control the patient's behavior are applied. There need not necessarily be any negligence on the part of the dentist, because catastrophic events do occur. Remember, there is no more sympathetic plaintiff than a mother of a child who was injured or died at the hands of a medical or dental care provider. Though possibly unfair, the general dentist who has an injury or medical mishap occur with a patient will find unjust criticism in the community and usually a lawsuit as a result.

Decide Whom You Will See

The first step to incorporating successful pediatric dentistry into a general practice is to have a clear policy regarding the decision criteria you use to determine which pediatric patients are appropriate for your skills, temperament, equipment, training and staff skills and training. When you have carefully determined all of your criteria, do not waver from the decision tree you have established. Once your criteria are established and operational for a period of time, practices and procedures that are beyond your routine referral methods are also now non-routine, and therefore bring a corresponding higher risk. To allow a parent or staff member talk you into attempting to treat a young patient when you have witnessed behaviors beyond those you have previously set as your referral criteria, is risking a potential disaster. If the procedure happens to go well, your criteria become less firm. Eventually you confront the limits of your ability and training, or in the case of a catastrophic event, that of your staff. If you get lucky, you refer a very difficult and risky patient to your friendly pediatric dentist who now must attempt to undo the damage. In any case, you erode your carefully planned protocols and your relationship with your pediatric dentist.

It's a bit like a pilot who flies deeper and deeper into the clouds, using rudimentary instrument flying skills learned in basic pilot training. As he successfully returns to the airport from these minor excursions in sightless flight, his confidence grows. Yet this is naked experience without training or instructor feedback, and it creates a growth of confidence that far exceeds the growth of skills. Soon the pilot ventures deeper and deeper into the clouds, flying on instruments without visual clues, and basing his decisions on the fact that he survived the last excursion. Often these pilots become a statistic when their confidence and memories of successful forays into dangerous territory leads to a final, deadly misadventure into unsuspected icing conditions.

Decide whom you will see in your practice, and stick with your decisions. If you decide to experiment on a patient using physical restraint or chemical sedation, then you are also experimenting with non-routine procedures and risk management.

In effect, the trusting patient and his family becomes "captive" to your decisions, because he relies on your professional judgment to determine which procedures are appropriate in your practice. The argument that patients are not truly at the doctor's mercy because they can choose another doctor, or see a pediatric dentist from the beginning, is simply not applicable in dentistry which as in all professions, is dedicated to holding the patient's well-being above that of the practitioner.

Communicate with Your Pediatric Dentist

Make sure your pediatric dentist knows your practice philosophy. As with all specialists, meet with him or her and discuss the guidelines you have determined for treatment planning in your practice, and see how they fit with the pediatric dentist's ideal. Like all other practitioners, the pediatric dentist would like to build a large and successful practice, and would like you to refer all your pediatric patients. They assert that their skills and training apply not only to taking care of management problems, but they should have the routine cases as well. There is some merit to these arguments, but enough common ground can be established to define when and where the appropriate referrals are made.

Whom to Refer

The pediatric dental practice is indispensable for certain categories of patients:

1. Medically compromised patients such as juvenile diabetics and hemophiliacs.
2. Developmentally disabled children who are unable to cope with the stresses of a dental visit.
3. Physically disabled children and adults who often feel better accommodation in a children's practice.
4. Children unable to cope with the stress of a dental visit and exhibit inappropriate coping mechanisms.
5. Sometimes for convenience of the family, and for valid behavioral reasons, the siblings of a referred patient.

Each of these may be a criterion in a given general practice. Make your own list, and then communicate your criteria first with your staff, then with the specialists.

Communication with the Parents and the Pediatric Dentist

Smooth referrals occur through excellent communication. It will require a meeting or series of meetings to interview perhaps several pediatric dentists, to choose one with whom you would like to work, and to work out the details of your referral communications. Once the relationship is established, then your attention can turn to the important protocols for communication with the parents or guardians of the patients who are to be referred. You can also inform your office management about these delicate relationships.

Parents often want their children to be seen in a single practice. Referring one child is a difficult event, especially for today's parents who have an almost compulsive desire to have "perfect" children. The report from a general dentist that little Sara's behavior is beyond the treatment capabilities of the general dental team is often alarming, and may even induce anger. It is important to use the best, most diplomatic and effective verbal skills to create a smooth and comfortable referral, and to send a happy and understanding parent to the pediatric dental visit. If the parent doesn't understand the need to have little Nathan referred, then she is often less accepting of the procedures used once they arrive at the specialist's practice.

The ideal standard office procedure is to see all patients for an initial examination, unless you routinely refer all children. Be careful not to create a *deferral* instead of a proper referral. A deferral occurs when a general dentist does not like to see very young children, but wants to see the slightly older ones. When this type of office is called, they report to the parents that children are not seen until age four, or whatever age the doctor prefers. In an uninformed parent, this is often interpreted to mean that there is *no need* for a small child to see a dentist, when nothing can be further from the truth. If you do not want to see very young children, be sure to properly inform the parents of your policy, and properly refer any new patients who are younger than your starting age.

When confronted for the first time with a dental visit, many small children will cry, but otherwise be cooperative. If no restorative needs are identified, the patient may be a candidate for continued care in the general practice. My personal recommendation is that if the child is under four years of age, and needs restorative work, then refer. If between age four and six, you might give a single attempt to perform the restorative procedure. If you are equipped with an air abrasion unit, and the restorations are suitable for conservative resins, then you should have a high rate of success. Otherwise, consider referral. After age five, most children can tolerate and accept most necessary procedures, including anesthesia and restorative procedures. If you have an uncooperative child in this age group, and cannot establish behavioral control easily in the first visit, then refer the patient to the pediatric dentist.

What do you tell the parent? First, be sure the doctor consults with the parent. He or she can be very specific with the description of the "difficult" behaviors without offending the parents. Communication from staff, though perfectly courteous and correct, may be offensive to parents when the subject is their child's behavior. At any rate, there is less debate from parents when the doctor makes the referral clear to the parent. The words must be carefully chosen. Phrases like "out of control," "behaved badly," or labels like "brat," "stubborn," or "obnoxious" have no place in oral communication or charting. Be very specific with the clinical reasons that treatment would be impossible.

Words to use are "won't open his mouth," "moves and struggles," "tries to fend the doctor off with his hands," "covers her mouth with her hands," "cries uncontrollably" and other terms that describe the situations. Often the parents have witnessed the events and are quite relieved that you have a solution. Tell the parent what the actions were that prevented you from getting the job done, and how it can add difficulty and risk to otherwise simple procedures. Then go on and inform them that Sonny can't be treated in this environment because he presents an "age-appropriate lack of cooperation more easily and appropriately handled in a pediatric practice." Always remain calm and reassuring; you are the professional. Don't back down when the parents try to prevail upon you to reconsider and try Sonny again. Simply tell them that there are procedures you have chosen not to provide, and consequently it would be beyond the training you have provided for your staff, and certainly outside of your routine. Making an exception would simply add unnecessary risk for the family. Don't be afraid to admit that there are procedures you choose not to do. Then offer words of confidence and encouragement about the pediatric practice. "He'll behave so well over there that you will wonder why we referred you!" Be positive and supportive, and complete the referral.

It is appropriate for a pediatric dentist to continue to treat a patient into his or her teens; many keep children in their practices to age 18. However, other pediatric dentists will refer the patient back at a specified age or simply after completion of restorative work. My preference is to have a cross-referral situation with my pediatric dentist whereby I refer only those patients I choose not to see, and leave the return referral up to the pediatric dentist. In return, I like to receive adult referrals from the pediatric dentist. Many parents will select a pediatric dentist out of the phone book or upon word of mouth referral, and establish a relationship for all the children in the family in that practice. The pediatric dentist should always inquire as to whom the referring dentist was, and hearing that there is none, should volunteer a referral for the parents. If you are not getting an occasional referral from your favorite pediatric dentist, ask why not. If it continues to be a one way street, then select a new pediatric dentist. A mutual referral network is neither illegal or unethical. It is simply good practice and good marketing, and is the least one professional can do for another whom he or she respects.

PEDIATRIC DENTAL COMMUNICATIONS

[pedocomm.14]

Desired Outcome: Identification and referral of appropriate patients to a pediatric dental practice so that the family understands and accepts the benefits of the referral and maintains the goodwill for the rest of the family in this practice.

Measurement: Patient will be identified as a referral candidate as early as possible in the relationship and will be referred without any failed treatment attempts.

1. Patient presents in office as a new patient or as an emergency.
2. Doctor meets parents and the patient and examines the patient. If the patient is cooperative during the examination, then continue attempts to get images and other records. If the patient cannot cooperate for the exam, consider going no further and refer.
3. Once a lack of cooperation is established, discontinue the exam.
4. Doctor consults with the patient to present and discuss benefits of pediatric dental referral.
5. **Pediatric Dental Referral Slip** is completed and signed by the doctor.
6. Doctor will call the pediatric dentist for a brief patient introduction. If doctor cannot call immediately, Patient Coordinator places the call. Patient coordinator places a telephone message in doctor's Telephone Return box to remind doctor to call the pediatric dentist for a brief consultation.
7. Doctor will call the pediatric dentist for a brief patient introduction.
8. Patient coordinator assists the patient in making an exam appointment at the office of the chosen pediatric dentist.

PEDIATRIC DENTAL REFERRAL SLIP

[pedoref.14]

Introducing:

Patient's Name ________________________________ Date _________
Address ____________________ City ____________ State ___ ZIP ____
Telephone _____________ FAX _______________ E-mail ____________

Medical history:

Dental history and treatment plan:

Reasons for referral; behavioral considerations:

Services requested; indicate teeth by description and location:

☐ Exam and treat circled teeth
☐ Referral for comprehensive care

1	2	3	4A	5B	6C	7D	8E	9F	10G	11H	12I	13J	14	15	16
32	31	30	29T	28S	27R	26Q	25P	24O	23N	22M	21L	20K	19	18	17

Special circumstances or requests; other specialists involved:

☐ Referral letter to follow

THANK YOU!

Signed ________________________________ D.D.S.

Chapter 15

IT'S OVER MY HEAD: COPING WITH THE COMPLEX PATIENT

"I'll never do another 'full mouth rehab' again!" Steve said emphatically.

"What was the problem with this one?" I asked.

"What wasn't?" Steve replied. "I might as well have married this patient, we have been seeing so much of each other!"

"Tell me about the case." I offered.

"Maggy seemed to be a case I could easily manage." Steve began. "She came in with the usual set of complaints for a person of her age, wanting to look better, to repair the broken down and shortened front teeth and get her general dental health in order. She was considering plastic surgery around her eyes and neck, so cosmetics was a big deal for her."

"But she also had major dental breakdown elsewhere?" I asked.

"Yes, very serious," Steve replied. "She had missing posterior teeth, and lots of wear facets and mobility. She was excellent with her oral hygiene, but still had redness and bleeding around her crowns, so she was afraid of getting more crowns done."

"Can't say as I blame her," I said. "It's difficult for patients to understand why they should get more restorations of a type that they feel contributed to their disease."

"Well, we developed a treatment plan and started in." In those days I was doing my own perio, such as it was, and we quickly got to the point where I could begin restorative. We completed ceramic restorations on the six upper front teeth, with margins right at the gingiva, so she was really happy with her appearance and gingival health," Steve reported.

"So you now had a motivated patient, ready for anything?" I commented.

"Yes, and she had the time and financial wherewithal to proceed." Steve began again, "She also was anxious to complete the dental treatment so she could get her face lift.

"Once we really got started, the trouble began. It seemed like every posterior tooth I prepared had postoperative discomfort. It was becoming a nightmare. As I worked my way around the arches, more and more complications arose. Soon, I was beginning to do root canals through some of my completed crowns, and I hadn't even finished the reconstruction," Steve lamented.

"Had you completed any occlusal analysis or occlusal therapy?" I queried.

"No." Steve was annoyed. "I really don't have a sufficient handle on vertical dimension to mess with opening a bite or anything likc that, and besides, I learned in school that you can seldom go wrong by preserving the vertical dimension and building your case in the acquired vertical. So I've completed all my cases that way since dental school. It seems to work most of the time. Where I get into trouble is cases like Maggy."

"What about the occlusal disease you observed? Do you believe that restoring in the 'acquired vertical dimension' would somehow correct the causes of the occlusal breakdown?" I asked.

"Well, yes. I was taught that the breakdown came from teeth shifting and becoming unstable from tooth loss," Steve replied. "We have brochures from the ADA that describe it just that way, and that's how I explain it to the patients."

"Using the brochures?"

"Yes, and other visual aids."

Steve went on: "Then more problems developed. The ceramic crowns began breaking down, fracturing and chipping. I decided that Maggy needed a night guard to protect the dental work. But, this did not sit well with Maggy. She had elected to do the case restoratively because she didn't want to have anything to do with orthodontics and really rebelled over the idea of a lifetime retainer. I could not get her to cooperate with any of my ideas or suggestions at this point."

"Had you lost her confidence?" I asked.

"Yes but we continued to work together for many more months, kind of on eggshells, until the case was completed," Steve said. "After that she wrote me a letter saying she was changing dentists. I'm still waiting for a letter or call from the next dentist."

"Are you anticipating problems?" I asked.

"The case never was right. I never got her to a point of comfort and completion. There was always a new problem popping up that interfered with our progress and needed immediate attention. Some of those situations were not entirely resolved when she left my practice. Plus she owes me a ton of money that I am afraid to try to collect," Steve said.

* * *

Steve's problems with Maggy are actually not rare or unique. This scenario is repeated daily in dental offices all over the country. As dental technology advances and patients become more aware of what we have to offer, they also become more sophisticated "consumers" of dental services. Cosmetic dentistry is a powerful marketing tool and the driving force of many practices. Patients are aware of a standard we have created that offers perfection in esthetics as a goal. Yet, many of these cases are in the condition they are in not because of caries or periodontal disease, but because of tooth wear from occlusal disease.

The "cosmetic dentists" who charge forward and restore the broken down anteriors with beautiful ceramic restorations, are often setting the stage for very serious complications in the not too distant future. To the trained eye, the elongation of incisors and cuspids that we see in cosmetic journals and alteration of the anterior guidance, which comes along for the ride, are serious mistakes that can only have negative results. The cause of the problem has not been addressed, and the forces that destroy enamel can more easily destroy dental ceramics or composites.

The solution is not a simple one, so I offer two stages. The first stage involves some careful introspection and an inventory of your actual skills to diagnose and treat occlusal problems. The second is to get the training you need to become the restorative dentist of the twenty-first century, not just some quick-fix artist of the past.

Dental schools do not adequately prepare students for the complex cases that we see today. People are living longer. Just as in medicine, where most of the diseases and conditions requiring treatment were not issues a few decades ago, dental needs of a population enjoying greater longevity are radically changing. Preservation of the dentition has brought challenges to the general practitioner that were seen by only a handful of elite practitioners in the immediate past. So the tools in the armamentarium of the typical general dentist do not comprise those necessary to examine, evaluate, diagnose and treat the complicated occlusal disease case. And before you reject this line of reasoning as immaterial because occlusal disease is rare, let me offer the conclusion held by most experience practitioners who treat occlusal disease: *Most adults have some elements of occlusal disease.* Fortunately, most do not also need full reconstruction.

The combination of early occlusal disease with only minor restorative needs has kept the average dentist out of trouble for many years. But, add "cosmetic" dentistry to the mix of services, and the time bomb just sped up. Alteration of anterior guidance without regard to centric relation will upset the homeostasis of many otherwise slowly progressing cases that were formerly without symptoms and turn the tide toward overt, symptomatic occlusal disease. The case gets out of control, and recovery is impossible without going back to the beginning and treating the occlusal problems. This is very difficult to do with a patient who was not educated and informed in the beginning of the need for occlusal therapy. Confidence is already nearly lost, and there is no way I know of to explain to a patient that you missed the most important element of his case in the initial exam and diagnosis, then expect him to stay with you for the recovery and do-over stages.

So, the first stage here is to refer the complex cases you encounter to a friend or colleague who has the skills "on the shelf" to complete the complex case. This is difficult for all of us to do. We're essentially admitting we are not capable of managing every case that comes our way. But it can also be a learning experience, and the colleague to whom you refer may be the mentor you need to learn to handle these cases yourself.

The second stage is to become very focused in your continuing education efforts for the next several years. It is nice to read the mail, and choose from a veritable supermarket of continuing education offerings that cross our desks daily. However, this "potpourri" approach does not lead to sustained, positive and measurable professional growth. It merely keeps us "informed." A better approach is to review your mission, and if it includes becoming a restorative dentist capable of handling all the complex restorative needs of your potential patients into the future, then consider an organized approach to learning the skills necessary to have "on the shelf" when the patients arrive.

My personal recommendation is to make a long-term commitment to attend the Pankey Institute for Advanced Dental Education, and complete the six Continuums offered there in four to five years. There you will learn all the skills necessary to provide complete therapy for most cases, including the complex cases involving occlusal disease, full mouth reconstruction, and the cases requiring advanced specialist cooperation such as we have been discussing in this book. You will learn to evaluate, diagnose, treatment plan, consult and treat the most challenging cases with confidence and success, on par with even the finest prosthodontists. Even the complex multidisciplinary case including advanced periodontal therapy and implants becomes a joy when all your doubts and concerns have been replaced with knowledge and skills. And it is a hands-on experience with clinical instructors who have been right where you are, in clinical practice making the tough decisions. The cost is reasonable. The benefits enormous.

There may be other ways to achieve the same result. But I have not seen any as direct, efficient and proven to provide measurable results in your practice.

The Local Prosthodontist

Your local prosthodontist is a great help in stage one, when you are referring the complex cases and acquiring the knowledge to treat them on your own. You will not find this to be a big practice builder; however, the new patients will likely become permanent patients in a modern prosthodontic practice that typically has a good hygiene program. Besides, would you want to be in a position to maintain the other doctor's work?

The prosthodontist *may* be a good mentor in your personal professional development. However, treat this relationship with caution, and evaluate the integrity and motivation of the prosthodontist to assist you in your professional growth. Your practice will ultimately be eliminated as a referral source for the prosthodontist, so unless you have a genuine personal friendship with the prosthodontist that precedes or goes far beyond your professional relationship, I believe this will be a mentoring trap that slows your progress. Even a well-meaning professional peer may take ten years or more to impart all the knowledge and experience that participation in the Pankey Continuums can achieve in a few short years.

But, do not hesitate to refer when necessary in the early stages of your path to clinical excellence. And do let the prosthodontist know what you are doing. It will keep the professional on his or her toes.

TMD Nightmares

Here again, referral may be necessary while you acquire the necessary skills to treat these cases. Much confusion and misinformation abound in this area, and many university continuing education courses leave the participants even more confused. It does not take a major research institute to diagnose and treat most cases of occlusal disease and TMD. It is a matter rather similar to the major complex restorative case, and many cases are the same individuals.

This is not a clinical instruction manual, so I will avoid any methodology for the assessment and treatment of TMD. However, it is again a matter of having the knowledge and skills in your repertoire in order to attract and treat the appropriate patients in a definitive manner. Initially, having a team of an excellent prosthodontist and oral surgeon to assist in your evaluation and treatment is imperative. Next, the curriculum at the Pankey Institute includes the areas of diagnosis and treatment planning for the TMD case.

The key to successful TMD treatment is successful patient communication and education. There is not always a definitive endpoint when TMD therapy begins, since therapeutic response varies, and treatment decisions are based upon those responses. Success is a comfortable patient, and there are lots of variations on the theme. Some patients will be in splint therapy indefinitely, others (hopefully most) will achieve an adaptive centric position to which they can be equilibrated and/or restored, with supportive splint therapy to continue at night in most cases. The essential skills for the doctor to possess are communication skills to enable the patient to understand the complexity of the case and its treatment and relationship skills to gain the patient's trust and compliance or agreement with therapy.

TMD cases are becoming more common in our population. The reasons are longevity of life, longevity of the dentition during life and stress of the post-modern world with all of its attending ill-health effects. The dentist of the future must have a working knowledge of the anatomy, biology, physiology and mechanics of the entire TM joint-occlusal system to be truly a physician of the head and neck.

Patient "Dumping"—The Specialist Perspective

Note that through all this discussion I have emphasized referral of cases where you are over your head in complexity or lack of armamentarium. From a specialist perspective, these cases may be a welcome addition to his or her practice. They may also be a problem of salvage for the referring doctor, even to the point of delicately avoiding a malpractice action against the referring doctor.

Patient "dumping," the almost-too-late referral of cases on the verge of failure is a problem throughout specialty practice. It is seldom discussed because of the nature of the referral relationship. Most specialists need your referrals to survive. When a general dentist initiates treatment, he or she is obligated to bring that therapy to a logical conclusion that meets the standard of care for that community. Most communities have an abundance of specialists, or there are specialists nearby, so the standard is quite simply that of a reasonable *specialist* in your community. If a doctor is unable to provide that level of therapy for the necessary recommended treatment, then it is his or her duty to refer. And in a timely manner.

Cases that are already failing are specially troublesome for the specialist. They must begin again to evaluate, diagnose, consult, plan treatment and initiate therapy with a patient who has "already been through this" with the referring doctor. Inevitably, the patient will raise the question of why all the examination, imaging, modeling and planning must occur again. It really puts the specialist on the spot. If he relies on data derived from your referral, and fails to find the appropriate diagnosis, then he risks clinical failure. If he chooses (rightfully) to begin again, then he must delicately address the issues of your competence—a question or concern the patient may raise.

It is in all of our best interests—patient, referring doctor, specialist, and dental community—to know our limitations and operate within them while seeking to expand the scope of our treatment ability. The only way I know to do this is to complete a comprehensive examination on all new patients and those with troubling new complaints. This includes mounted study models on all cases with any single sign of occlusal disease. Then, it is simple to take a look at the data, and even consult with a mentor or specialist before making any treatment decisions and therapeutic commitment to the patient. Intercepting those patients who have problems that are unable to be resolved within the current scope of your own skills, and perhaps meeting briefly in advance with a specialist to get some ideas about the case makes you, the dentist, look profoundly competent. Case presentations are clear and the referral is a seamless effort to gain the best results for the patient without any embarrassing retreat.

Ours is truly a complex and demanding profession. It takes enormous expertise and intellect to treat the scope of potential problems that enter the doors of the typical modern dental practice. The necessary skills are barely introduced in dental school, and only a planned concerted effort by the most committed practitioners in the area of continuing education will result in mastery of the skills necessary to treat the complex case in a comprehensive manner. Those proficiencies include behavioral, social or relationship, and communication skills, as well as management and technical skills. All of these skills are integrated into the curriculum in the six Continuums of the L.D. Pankey Institute for Advanced Dental Education. While acquiring the skills necessary for clinical mastery, dentists need excellent working relationships with their patients, staffs and specialists. Referrals are best made early, after careful comprehensive examination and diagnosis has taken the patient out of the realm of the doctor's current skill set and before therapy is initiated.

COMPLEX CASE COMMUNICATIONS

[compcom.15]

Desired Outcome: Successful comprehensive treatment from case identification and referral to case completion. Patient will not remain a patient of this practice, but will proceed in another practice to planning completion of the comprehensive treatment plan. Patient may return for hygiene care later, though the trend in most prosthodontic and advanced general practices is to retain the patients for future care and follow-up.

Measurement: Ninety percent of cases referred accept treatment recommendations; 100 percent of cases initiated go to completion.

1. Case is identified by doctor as a complex referral.
2. Study models, images and the patient record are provided for doctor to initiate case study.
3. Initial diagnosis and treatment planning are completed, with resultant realization of complex requirement's beyond current capabilities.
4. Consultation is scheduled by patient coordinator with the patient: to discuss and present benefits of referral.
5. **Complex Case Referral Slip** is completed and signed by the doctor.
6. Patient coordinator places a telephone message in doctor's Telephone Return box to remind doctor to call the prosthodontist.
7. Doctor will call the prosthodontist for a brief patient introduction.
8. Patient coordinator assists the patient in making an exam appointment at the office of the chosen doctor.
9. Patient coordinator schedules a pretreatment consultation between the doctors.

Complex Case Communications / 2

10. Doctor will meet quarterly with the prosthodontist to discuss cases in progress. This is necessary to know the outcomes of cases you have referred.
11. Patient coordinator will track all cases in progress and note cases nearing completion on the Complex Case Patient Monitor. Report this during the morning huddle.
12. Doctor will send a small thank you note to the prosthodontist in response to his case completion letter.

COMPLEX CASE REFERRAL SLIP

[compcase.15]

Introducing:

Patient's Name ______________________________ Date __________
Address ____________________ City ____________ State ____ ZIP _____
Telephone _____________ FAX _______________ E-mail _____________

Medical history:

Dental history and treatment plan:

□ See attached initial treatment plan

Services requested:

Special circumstances or requests; other specialists involved:

□ Referral letter to follow
□ Case planning meeting requested

THANK YOU!

Signed __________________________________ D.D.S.

SAMPLE REFERRAL LETTER

[sampref.15]

JAY M. HISLOP, D.D.S.

Excellence in Dentistry

Gerry Bowman, D.D.S.
2231 Amber Drive
Stockton, CA 95299

Dear Gerry:

SUBJECT: RHONDA DONNER

This letter is to introduce Rhonda Donner to your practice. Rhonda is a 41-year-old female who presented to our office for initial examination with the following:

- Moderate to locally advanced periodontitis.

- Numerous broken down alloy and direct composite restorations.

- Signs of wear and occlusal breakdown including cervical abfractions, posterior wear facets and anterior crossover facets.

- Symptoms of TMD including the following: Trigger point pain, headaches, limitation upon opening, bilateral early reciprocal clicks, a 1mm slide CO-CR. Please refer to occlusal exam record enclosed.

Gerry Bowman, DDS, p. 2

• Her goals for treatment are to look beautiful and feel more comfortable. She is a very attractive woman, but her worn anteriors and visibly darkened restorative work are cosmetic problems that definitely detract from her appearance. She is frustrated that no dentist has ever resolved these problems satisfactorily, and she cannot do anything about them herself.

• She has expressed to Judy, our patient coordinator, that this is a high priority at this time in her life, and has presented no barriers to treatment, other than some minor scheduling requests.

We have completed our initial exam and concluded:

• Periodontal evaluation revealed need for initial periodontal therapy and possibly mucogingival surgery with grafts in three quadrants.

• Occlusal disease is present and advanced.

• TMJ's are not stable. Occlusal muscle symptoms are present.

• Teeth # 3, 4, 8, 9, 11, 15, 18, 27, 30, 31 are seriously challenged. There are edentulous spaces which the patient would like evaluated for implants.

Our anticipated treatment plan is:

1. Referral for periodontal comprehensive care.
2. Completion of comprehensive implant/restorative care in your office.
3. Follow-up care in your office.
4. As always, I would like a final case presentation for my own learning and communication.

Gerry Bowman, DDS, p. 3

Would you please examine Rhonda and have Christine make arrangements with Lisa for our pre-treatment consultation?

Thanks for your help with this interesting and challenging case.

Sincerely,

Jay M. Hislop, D.D.S.

JH:ct

Chapter 16

SAYING GOODBYE: NOT ALL RELATIONSHIPS ARE FOREVER

"So I could have handled Maggy a lot differently!" Steve admitted.

"When would you have let her go if you could do it over again?" I asked.

"Probably right after the initial exam, except I'm still not sure how I would have known," Steve said. "But now I understand from experience that even minor signs of occlusal disease can manifest as major symptoms when the dentist intervenes with as much change as I created in Maggy's case. I really want to learn how to handle the cases better clinically. In the meantime, I need to manage the relationships better."

Saying Goodbye

There are four categories of patients that a dentist might have occasion to release from the practice.

The first and most obvious are those patients who decide to leave. These may be patients who are moving to a distant community or those leaving for another local practice. In each case, the patient coordinator should contact the patient and conduct an exit interview to establish the level of satisfaction the patient experienced in the practice. It is essential because it might benefit the ones remaining in the community. Some may be leaving because of insurance changes to a closed panel HMO or DMO, coupled with low patient dental IQ and low value placed by the patient upon dental care. But others may be genuinely dissatisfied. If so, it is important to conduct a satisfaction interview to (1) determine the patient's reason for leaving the practice, and (2) establish a positive, final contact with the patient that will often diffuse their anger, and leave them less likely to communicate their displeasure with others.

The second category of patients you may need to say goodbye to are those who are *"financial promise breakers."* These are the patients who fail consistently to keep their financial obligations to the practice. Though I do not recommend a policy that allows credit to be extended for dental services, it is necessary in some cases to get a patient moving along through an acute phase of treatment. By the time definitive restorative treatment is to be recommended in a consultation, the financial issues of the patient should have already been resolved, and his or her commitment to dental treatment is high, making the financial arrangement less of an issue for the practice. At that stage, most patients will have identified a personal source of funds to pay for the treatment, so it will not be the doctor's responsibility to finance the treatment. But there still are those few patients who fail to meet a simple financial obligation like an insurance copayment.

The third category of patients are those with unrealistic expectations and numerous negative perceptions of dentistry that the doctor and dental staff are unable to overcome prior to initiating treatment. These may be the patients with whom you just cannot seem to communicate. That is not to say they are unreasonable or combative, but they merely trigger a personality conflict that makes your blood pressure rise. The blessing is they usually know it as well and may be struggling with a solution themselves. These patients are the chronic complainers whom you cannot please, no matter your effort. They must be carefully distinguished from the discerning patient who demands *and appreciates* your very best services and attention. The former you may want to release, the latter you are trying to attract.

Finally, in the fourth category are those patients for whom your skill set is inappropriate. An example is the difficult restorative case for Maggy, discussed in the previous chapter.

In each of these cases, the goals are to release the patient from the practice; to see that they are referred for specialty care, if appropriate; to communicate the options for further care available for the patient; to preserve patient goodwill in the community; and to eliminate the possibility of accusations of abandonment.

PATIENT RELEASE FROM PRACTICE

[release.16]

Desired Outcome: Successful patient release from the practice will be accomplished when a patient has been referred to another office for comprehensive care, whether a geographically distant office, or a local specialty restorative practice with preservation of goodwill and no risk of patient abandonment.

Measurement: Doctor is satisfied that he is working primarily with compatible patients, and no cases abandoned.

1. Case is identified by doctor as a candidate for release, or the patient informs the practice of an impending move to another city or another local practice.
2. The patient is contacted by the patient coordinator.
3. An exit interview is conducted for those patients who inform the practice that they are leaving. The purpose is to politely determine the reasons that the patient is leaving the practice.
4. If the patient is being released by the doctor, this is best managed in writing, through the mail. After receiving the letter, the patient may call in, and the exit interview may be conducted at that time.
5. **Patient release** is documented in the patient's clinical record, including referral recommendations and conversations with the patient.

Patient Release from Practice / 2

6. Patient records are immediately copied and prepared for collection by the patient, and stored in the records storage area awaiting the patient's arrival. This prevents embarrassing encounters in the reception area should an angry patient have to wait for records.
7. Patients are to receive their most current X-rays, study models, medical history, dental and periodontal charting and billing records. Progress notes and treatment plans are not to be copied and given unless subpoenaed.
8. A sample release letter follows.

Sample Release Letter: The following letter is appropriate for the patient who is moving.

JAY M. HISLOP, D.D.S.

Excellence in Dentistry

Gerry Lester
1221 Stardust Drive
Stockton, CA 95299

Dear Gerry:

SUBJECT: CONTINUED DENTAL CARE

It has been a pleasure to be of service to you for the last __ years. We hope that as you move on with your life that you find satisfactory dental services in your new location. If we can be of any assistance in that effort, please let us know. We have contacts in various communities around the nation and may be of some assistance as you seek to establish professional relationships in your new location.

Please stop by the office before you leave to pick up a copy of your most recent X-rays and a portfolio that includes your study models and records. Call Katy a few days in advance so she can have that ready for you.

We'll sure miss your smile around here!

Sincerely,

JH:ct

Jay M. Hislop, D.D.S.

Sample Release Letter: For patients the doctor chooses to release. This may seem a bit cold, but it is necessary to prevent legal action.

J A Y M . H I S L O P , D . D . S .

E x c e l l e n c e i n D e n t i s t r y

Gerry Lester
1221 Stardust Drive
Stockton, CA 95299

Dear Gerry:

SUBJECT: CONTINUED DENTAL CARE

I am no longer able to continue as your dentist because _______________ (insert any one of the following, or other rational and logical reason. Note, no reason at all need be given):

- of your failure to make an effort to pay for dental services.
- of your failure to comply with treatment recommendations.
- of your failure to make and keep dental appointments.
- of our mutual inability to form and maintain a working profcssional relationship.

Mr. Gerry Lester, p. 2

I urge you to seek the services of another dentist as soon as possible. To assist you in that endeavor, you may contact the dental referral service of the local dental society at 111-1111.

You may come by the office at any time to collect your most recent X-rays and study models. Please call an hour in advance so Katy can have those ready for you.

(You may add the following paragraph, but it is not required):

I will be available for emergency services only for a period of 30 days from the date of this letter. Thereafter, you will need to have made arrangements for continued dental care in another office.

Sincerely,

Jay M. Hislop, D.D.S.

JH:ct

Chapter 17

AFTER THE INK DRIES: KEEPING THE DREAM ALIVE

A Working Document

All the effort of practice design and planning, continuing education and relationship building is wasted if business continues as usual. All of a premier dental practice's mission, procedures and concepts must be written down and shared among the staff. It becomes a training tool and a review program for staff meetings.

One of the most important, underrated and underutilized reasons for a complete set of documents that include the mission and procedures of a dental practice is the preservation of the value of the practice at time of transition, disability or death of the doctor. If the practice has proven that it is capable of weathering a recession or two, has been able to easily train new staff members, has incorporated temporary staff members into the daily routine immediately and seamlessly, it has much greater value to a prospective partner or buyer.

Documentation also allows for ease of adjustment to future changes. Dentistry is anything but static, and changes are expected to be more rapid and of greater amplitude in the near future. Change is difficult, if not impossible, when there is no foundation of understanding of the present working conditions. Conversely, when the current operating methods and rational for them are documented, understood and used as a weekly training tool, change is a simple matter.

The process looks something like this: A new pressure is placed upon a practice, say a rapidly changing technology of recent years such as intraoral video. The doctor and the staff are not sure how the new technology will fit into their practice. They see the demonstrations at the conventions, and it looks good, but cannot imagine how to fit it into their routine. They do not even know if they need to consider incorporating it. But if the practice has mission and a set of standard operating procedures, they can look to those for guidance. Perhaps the doctor is already using a 35mm camera, and the protocols would allow the introduction of video at certain stages of the new patient exam. The hygiene routine may be reviewed, and the use of video may be considered as a time saver for patient education. Communications with specialists are reviewed, and the video camera is able to provide direct video communications with one of the selected specialists, with whom the office already communicates with on line. The appropriate procedures are conditionally updated, and a staff meeting is held to discuss the feasibility and to demonstrate the actual application of the new technology in specific ways in this practice *before the salesman even gets an invitation to come and demonstrate the technology!*

Updates and EDITS

It is a continuous process to review, reconsider, update, and edit the entire scope of the dental practice from mission and standard operating procedures through patient and specialist communications. Once the original documents are in place, updating these protocols will be relatively easy. It will help create a practice that is entirely prepared for the rapid changes we all now face. This foundation prepares the practice to plan and act in advance in the face of changing business conditions, and to respond quickly and efficiently to unexpected changes. If you don't know where you are or precisely what you are doing, how can you possibly plan and execute appropriate changes? Written communication documents and formats create the foundation for confident action. The alternative—action without direction—inevitably leads to greater chaos.

Periodic Specialist Meetings

Keeping abreast of changes in the specialties is easy if you are in continuous dialog with your selected specialists. Let each of them know that you are interested in detailed and current information about the technology and procedures that they have available, to better enable you to appropriately plan treatment. It is a good idea to meet periodically to discuss pending cases, cases in progress and completed case outcomes. Specialists often do not have a clear perspective on their results, since the patients are referred back to the general practice for continuing care. Be sure to bring evidence of the successful treatment outcomes to each meeting so that the specialist gets a sense of his or her contribution. Also discuss the less than desired results. Though more difficult to approach, the subjects of failed or less than hoped for results are important considerations for future case planning.

Bring the results of those meetings back to the practice, and use the information to keep your communication documents in state-of-the-art format for your specialists. This will impress them with your knowledge and ability, and motivate them to give you the very best they have to offer in service and information. Everybody wins.

Like any other life endeavor, successful dental practice is really the creation of good habits, which are supported and repeated. When communication of your mission becomes a habit that is exemplified by all of your daily actions, relationships and services, you cannot fail to achieve the practice of your dreams.

Epilogue

A DAY ON THE BAY

It was a startlingly bright morning in February. The cold wind was steady through the Golden Gate. Reflections of the mid-morning sun danced on the surface of the swells like silver coins. Steve's boat, a 36-foot sloop, had rounded Alcatraz Island and was heeled slightly over on a gentle port reach aiming for Tiburon. The sails seemed solid. Flexible fabric turned into giant unmoving walls of wind towering above our heads, the uncontrolled power of the wind harnessed by design and expert hands. Sails transform when aloft. From the dark wrinkled repose of a bag below, they spring to life and provide an unbelievably smooth and brilliant engine for the vessel. The sailboat sliced the rolling swells, showering us occasionally with a light but very cold spray. We looked like fisherman from the wharf or America's Cup competitors in our yellow slickers and black deck boots.

I felt quite relaxed and comfortable, but Steve was concerned for my well-being. He'd become a veteran of many such days on the bay in the last two years, and was used to, even drawn to the harsh conditions. I was his guest, experiencing the elements he had once only dreamed about.

"You doing all right?" Steve asked.

"I'm fine," I replied. "This is a spectacular day, and I can't think of a better way to enjoy it!"

"It keeps me going," Steve said. "I find that my time on the water seems to help me focus so well that it gives me back more time on land. Does that make any sense?"

"Sure it does!" I replied. "The duties and responsibilities of our lives—the practice, the patients, our families, providing dental care, working with staff can only become a joy when a doctor has a balanced life."

"And has his values in order and his systems under control," Steve added.

"Exactly, and you've done a marvelous job since we began our work together," I offered.

"It's not hard for me to remember exactly how it was in those days. And I remember how it felt. I'd only dream about days like this on the water. I recall the frustration of not really feeling like I was making a contribution to my patients or my family. I remember the feeling of overwhelming debt, my personal fitness was out of control, and the staff seemed like they were just putting in time to the end of the day," Steve recalled.

"It seemed like I was making no progress toward my goals when I realized I really didn't have any true goals, only vague mental images of something. Taking inventory of my values and writing a mission has been far more important in my life than I believed it would be when you coached me through the process."

"That's not a surprise to me," I said. "Most people never take the time or don't know how to establish the philosophical foundations for a lifetime of happiness and fulfillment. It seems like too tall of an order. It's hard to map unknown territory. Yet the best lives are those lived with intention and self-awareness. And personal direction and leadership that really emotionally grabs and inspires you."

"That really is what it takes," Steve agreed. "My practice has gone places in two short years that I would never have believed possible when I began this process. I have so much to be thankful for today."

"Tell me about that," I asked.

Steve took his eyes off the horizon for a moment to look directly at me. He smiled and his shoulders relaxed as he corrected slightly on the helm.

"All right. I am thankful that I now have a practice that has a heart, a spirit of its own. It is larger than I am. Larger than the sum of my staff and me," Steve began.

"This practice provides something for patients I never dreamed of. My staff and I are in such alignment with our values and our mission that we are able to form relationships with our patients that are truly harmonious. There are very few conflicts in the office. We have our differences, but the staff crosses over those differences with compassion and forbearance. They really work hard on solutions to the problems we face. I never believed any workplace could be so meaningful to both the people who work there and the people whom we serve. Every person on my staff is trying to make a positive impact on the patients every day. The patients have come to know and feel this as well."

Steve paused. "Am I an 'Eagle'?" he asked.

"And more," I replied. "You see, the strata of dental practices is really based upon economics. It is a way to see how a practice stacks up when compared to others in the nation. But the system has its limits. Your practice is now on economically sound footings, and it has become something more than just an 'Eagle' practice. Your practice is now a mature business entity that operates on a much higher philosophical and managerial plane than most other practices. Your business is run from a set of personal values that are translated through your mission to become a relationship-based business instead of the old style transaction-based business. People don't come to you because you offer a service, a single transaction or chain of transactions. Crowns and fillings are commodities. They come to you because they seek health and comfort, dignity and beauty. They believe they can trust you and your staff to have the character and wisdom to treat them in their personal best interest. They want to form a relationship of trust and respect with someone of good character and reputation who they believe acts with wisdom to provide what is best for them. They know your network of associations with specialty practices is also designed to provide the best for the patient.

"I suspect there are many personal milestones for you as well," I added.

"Yes. I spend a great deal of time with examination and treatment planning because it is important for me to know my patients. This makes my case presentations more comprehensive, and I don't worry much about case acceptance. The patients seem to trust in what I am offering them and generally want to follow my plan. The specialists are all in alignment with my plans and the patients feel that too." Steve replied.

"I also spend far less time on management issues, though it took a lot of time and effort to get it that way. We now deal with things as they arise and the staff takes the initiative to redesign the procedures in ways they feel are more effective and efficient. They feel important and involved in the process. They also know that they can have a definite and positive impact on their workplace. It all gets reduced to a written procedure and placed in the manual after we meet and discuss the solutions. It's just a weekly event now and nobody thinks very much of it. It is routine."

The wind shifted slightly and the sails began to luff. Rather than drop down to port on the whim of the wind, Steve gave a couple of quick commands and we came about. I hauled in the jib sheet while Steve tended the mainsail. The sails filled and the boat seemed to jump from the water as it accelerated on a new starboard tack headed toward Fort Point. The sun back lit the sails; they seemed to glow with an internal luminescence.

Steve continued: "I am much more relaxed and comfortable now. This staff has never seen the anger and frustration I used to project to my former employees. I now realize how much of the problem was not with the staff, but with me. I have more time in the office to practice dentistry, and I spend my unscheduled time for pre-treatment planning and building staff relationships.

"I get out the door on time at the end of the day, and I am anxious to get to work in the morning. My attitude is a thousand percent improved. I have the time to think and reflect on how things are going. The staff takes my input very seriously and acts upon my suggestions rapidly. Of course, they are able to bring their knowledge and skill to every problem, so my solution is not always the one we use. But they are very respectful of my input and comments.

"Surprisingly, the office is very light-hearted and fun!" Steve said.

"Why is that a surprise?" I asked.

"Well, I would have thought that with all this values-based planning, with the several missions and practice philosophy and very formal communication and standardized work structures that we would feel quite regimented in our approach to each day."

"And what did you find?" I asked.

"We are so well organized that it doesn't feel regimented at all. We all know what to do so procedures and communications with patients and between our specialty offices are seamless. This leaves us a lot of valuable time to spend getting to know our patients and each other. The organization has freed us to do our work well and be ourselves in relationships with our patients and each other. The tone of the office is very professional but also very warm. It is a fun and happy place to spend some time. That is truly a surprise to me!

"Obviously, I have achieved my goal of being able to sail more. I now am on the water at least two times a week. I started hanging around the sailing club again and now have some racing buddies. We finished second in the Wednesday Regatta last week on a friend's boat. It is really great to be active again."

"You look like you're in better shape too," I commented.

"Yes. I've dropped 16 or 17 pounds. My exercise program is somewhat more focused, but the real reason is I don't eat for comfort anymore. My life is good so I can control my eating habits. I used to eat late at night just to settle down.

"And my family has begun to get used to having me around the house! I am so much more involved with my family, the kids' activities and all. Not quite to the level of 'Mr. Mom,' but I really wasn't aware of how much I was missing," he added. "My family has begun to include me in things that they didn't bother even asking about before, like helping with homework and spontaneous trips to the movies or a game of catch."

"My wife and I have been able to take more time to get to know each other all over again. Raising a family becomes such a focus that you lose sight of each other. We still have days that go by without much meaningful time together, but we are pretty cautious about not letting too many days pass without taking time for each other, to talk and visit about how things are going."

"How much time are you spending in the office?" I asked.

"Well, here's a surprise. I'm spending five days in the office, actually more than before, but they are more normal work days. I see patients four days and sometimes an extra half day. Otherwise I spend the 'extra' half day or whole work day organizing my systems, planning cases, and all the things I used to do in the late evenings or at home," he answered.

"So you spend more hours in the office?" I clarified.

"Probably more days, but the same total hours," Steve replied. "But again, my time there is more productive. And the organization we're able to accomplish on my administrative and planning days really allows for far greater efficiency on clinical days. The end result is I am spending time at the office but freeing my remaining time from any office-related activities. I feel like I have better balance and my family confirms it."

"So is it perhaps misguided for dentists to try to achieve the elusive three-and-a half day work week?" I asked.

"In my case, yes," Steve replied. "I have truly more free time for my family and my sailing than I ever had when I was trying for the short work week. I plan ahead for the afternoons that I sail. We have one evening a week that we see patients. This frees an entire morning for me. I work one Saturday per month to see one or two comprehensive-care patients for major treatment. But when I leave the office, my time is truly my own. I really love the way I feel now. Both enthusiastic commitment when I'm there and total freedom from it when I'm not. I look forward to going into the office now. We're doing better financially too."

We sailed into Tiburon where we docked and had some lunch. It was a perfect day.

Steve's story is not an illusion. It is a dream that can be achieved by any dentist willing to take the steps and pay the price in time and introspection. The effort required is not insurmountable, but it is significant. The payoff is enormous. Why should you settle for anything less?

INDEX—Designing Your Perfect Dental Practice

G

H

I

J

L

M

N

O

P